REIKI

Self Empowerment Guide to Reiki Healing & Reiki Meditation

(Learn Reiki and Crystal Techniques to Increase Your Energy and Master Self- Healing Techniques to Reduce Stress and Anxiety)

Steve Rand

Published by Rob Miles

Steve Rand

All Rights Reserved

Reiki: Self Empowerment Guide to Reiki Healing & Reiki Meditation (Learn Reiki and Crystal Techniques to Increase Your Energy and Master Self- Healing Techniques to Reduce Stress and Anxiety)

ISBN 978-1-989990-48-3

All rights reserved. No part of this guide may be reproduced in any form without permission in writing from the publisher except in the case of brief quotations embodied in critical articles or reviews.

Legal & Disclaimer

The information contained in this book is not designed to replace or take the place of any form of medicine or professional medical advice. The information in this book has been provided for educational and entertainment purposes only.

The information contained in this book has been compiled from sources deemed reliable, and it is accurate to the best of the Author's knowledge; however, the Author cannot guarantee its accuracy and validity and cannot be held liable for any errors or omissions. Changes are periodically made to this book. You must consult your doctor or get professional medical advice before using any of the suggested remedies, techniques, or information in this book.

Upon using the information contained in this book, you agree to hold harmless the Author from and against any damages, costs, and expenses, including any legal fees potentially resulting from the application of any of the information provided by this guide. This disclaimer applies to any damages or injury caused by the use and application, whether directly or indirectly, of any advice or information presented, whether for breach of contract, tort, negligence, personal injury, criminal intent, or under any other cause of action.

You agree to accept all risks of using the information presented inside this book. You need to consult a professional medical practitioner in order to ensure you are both able and healthy enough to participate in this program.

Table of Contents

INTRODUCTION 1

CHAPTER 1: HISTORY OF YOGA 3

CHAPTER 2: THE FIRST CHAKRA 8

CHAPTER 3: TYPES OF REIKI AND OTHER HEALING (INFO FOR ADVANCED STUDENTS ONLY) 14

CHAPTER 4: REIKISELF-TREATMENTS 44

CHAPTER 5: THE HISTORY OF ANGELS 74

CHAPTER 6: THE BENEFITS OF REIKI 80

CHAPTER 7: THE PRINCIPLES OF REIKI 87

CHAPTER 8: REIKI AND BUDDHISM 99

CHAPTER 9: THE IMPORTANCE OF INITIATION SIZE 106

CHAPTER 10: DAILY REIKI PRACTICE 130

CHAPTER 11: HOW TO PRACTISE REIKI AFTER ATTUNEMENT 142

CHAPTER 12: INTRODUCING YOU TO BEGINNER YOGA EXERCISES 147

CHAPTER 13: LIVING WITHOUT WORRY 151

CHAPTER 14: SUPREME PRECEPTOR 167

CONCLUSION 190

Introduction

The essence of chakras is that everything within the body can be healed. It starts with the inner voice telling you that something is wrong. If you don't heed that inner voice, your emotions will tell you that something is wrong in your consciousness. If you still don't heed your emotions, symptoms will begin to show in your physical body. Ultimately, you like everyone else want to be happy. If you want to be happy, you must ensure that your chakras are balanced.

This book is intended for beginners who want to learn about chakras and how they can take advantage of it. By reading this book, it is the hope of the writer that you learn and are encouraged to practice the balancing of the chakras in order to have a healthy and balanced life.

Thanks again for downloading my book, I hope you enjoy it!

Chapter 1: History Of Yoga

The practice of yoga dates back to the Indus Valley civilization (around 2600 - 1900 BCE). Early Buddhist texts, Upanishads, and even the Bhagavad Gita, all have mentions of yoga in them. To follow something without knowing its origin is of no use.

The latest archeological evidence of yoga is found in around 3000 B.C but there are traces of evidence to believe that it was practiced even before that i.e. about 5000 years ago. Initially it started as a community oriented tradition and later got transformed as an individual's convention. The history of yoga is divided into four phases:

Vedic period

Pre-classical period

Classical period

Modern period

Vedic Period

Vedas that are the sacred guide of Brahmanism that is practiced now as Hinduism in the modern period, has the yoga teachings in the form of ceremonies and rituals. These ceremonies and rituals helped the people to live their life in divine peace.

Pre-Classical period

Here, Upanishads mark the existence of yoga. There are around 200 scriptures that talk about the instinct of foreseeing a situation resulting from adherence of a discipline. They explain about the final reality (Brahman), The Spiritual self (Atman) and the relation between the two.

Yoga was a practice not only associated with Hinduism; evidences state that these were also followed in Buddhism through "Meditation" which is an important part of yoga.

Classical period

Second century marked the standardization of Yoga through a creation named "Yoga Sutra" by Patanjali. Being considered as the father of yoga, his book influences the modern yoga in many ways. The entire yoga is organized in his book in a systematic approach. Yoga here, is divided into eight limbs; giving the ways and means to attain ecstasy i.e. Samadhi.

The eight limbs are:

YAMA – Ethical values

NIYAMA – Observance

ASANAS – Exercises

PRANAYAMA – Breath regularization

PRATYAHARA - Abstraction/Withdrawal

DHARANA – Talks about concentration

DHYANA – Meditation

SAMADHI – Enlightenment

Modern period

This is about the 1800 and 1900 where yoga attained popularity as the masters started to draw attention and admirers who started following what they practiced through immense travel which started from west.

In the time between the classical and modern period yoga masters created an organized system to be followed to achieve ecstasy. In this process they denied the preaching of the Vedas and

Upanishads, thereby focusing on present. Here physical body is considered as a means to achieve Samadhi.

Here the focus is shifted to understand, accept and live the situation for understanding of the final reality.

There were many recognized gurus like Swami Vivekananda, Swami Siva Nanda (who gave the five principles of yoga), Maharishi Mahesh (the follower of Transcendental meditation) and more.

The ways and means opted by various gurus might be different, but they all point toward the same general direction of well-being and healthy lifestyle.

Chapter 2: The First Chakra

Now that you understand the basic concepts that explain what chakras are and how they function, you are ready to study how individuals such as yourself can open the seven main chakras, recharge them and use them for vital energy and inner peace. This chapter will discuss the first or root chakra.

Earth Chakra

The first chakra is located at the base of our spine and is the entry point of the earth's energy into our bodies. The first chakra is important because without it, no energy from the earth and its creatures could ever enter our bodies. In Sanskrit, the earth chakra is home to the Kundalini or the coiled serpent. This serpent is said to represent all that is primal in a human-most important of which is the need for survival.

The first chakra is controls the horizontal section of the body just below the sexual organs. It affects the digestion and excretion of food, as well as the instincts that have helped our race progress and grow. This chakra is often blocked by the emotion we call fear. It is also associated with the color red. Without the first chakra you will not be able to feel a deep connection with the earth that nourishes you, nor will you be able to understand that everything is connected to each other. This is why it is important to open and recharge this chakra point first, before moving on to the others.

Opening the earth chakra

To open the earth or first chakra, you must first recognize and name your fears. What are your fears? Who do you fear? What circumstances or events do you fear? You must be honest with yourself. Once you realize what your fears are, you will be able to give them proper faces. These faces you place on your fears will help you see that they are, in fact, nothing to fear. You will learn that most of what you hold as frightening are illusions or misunderstandings you have made yourself believe.

Let go of these fears. Surrender them to the universe, and let the energy from your first chakra flow from the earth, to your feet, your lower limbs, and pool at the base of your spine. Release your fears and welcome the energy of the earth.

Physical exercises to open and recharge the earth chakra

The earth or root chakra is related to all the physical activities of the body. This is because all physical movement is not possible without coming into contact with the earth or ground. Some people who have successfully opened their first chakra engaged in the martial arts to strengthen their lower limbs, and literally feel the earth under their feet as they moved and practiced formations. However, if you choose to strengthen your earth chakra this way, remember that exhaustion drains the chakra point, and is not healthy for the body. You must remember to strike a balance between strengthening your body for the earth chakra, and driving it to the point of exhaustion.

Two simple exercises to recharge the earth chakra

There are two simple exercises you can do every day in order to keep your earth chakra open, and recharge it at the same time. The first exercise is called grounding.

Step 1: Stand up straight and maintain a relaxed position. Your feet must be bare. If you can go outside and stand on soil, then that would be much better.

Step 2: Move your feet sideways until they are separated by the width of your shoulders.

Step 3: Close your eyes. Bend your knees slowly. Keep your breathing calm and even.

Step 4: Move your hips slightly forward, so that your weight is balanced on the soles of your feet.

Step 5: Focus your body's weight on your feet. Inhale and exhale slowly. Imagine energy travelling from the soil, and entering through your feet. Feel that energy give you its strength. Hold this position for at least two minutes. Repeat as often as you can.

The second exercise is much simpler and can be done even if you are seated at work or in school. This exercise is called contracting.

Step 1: Whether you are seated or standing, begin by monitoring your breathing. Be sure to take even, deep breaths until your entire body is calm.

Step 2: Focus on the base of your spine, and the area that the earth chakra controls.

Step 3: Contract the muscles of your bottom to stimulate the anus and the genitals, in order to send energy flowing into the earth chakra.

Step 4: Inhale deeply, and contract the muscles as in step 3.

Step 5: Exhale slowly, and relax your muscles.

Repeat steps 4 and 5 as often as possible, for at least two minutes every day.

You can also recharge your earth chakra by eating root crops such as potatoes, carrots, onions and beets.

Chapter 3: Types Of Reiki And Other Healing (Info For Advanced Students Only)

There are different types of Reiki (and other forms of healing). They are all taught differently and have individual techniques, but the general principles are similar. I have put these types of Reiki into categories, although some may overlap. There are also other forms of Reiki and healing that I haven't included.

There is a debate as to whether these different types of healing use the same energy and frequencies. Most people (including myself) can feel different types of energy with the different systems, but it is possibly different aspects of the same energy. It is also believed by some that healing and energies exist on different levels e.g. levels 1-7, some believe 352 levels.

Why are there different schools of Reiki? Basically, there are different schools of Reiki because students have gone on to add their own ideas and develop new techniques. As well as Reiki, there are also other forms of healing that exist throughout history. Some of these have influenced Reiki, whilst some are completely separate.

It is up to you which school or schools you follow. Do your research first and respect other traditions.

POPULAR WESTERN VARIATIONS ON USUI REIKI

USUI SHIKI RYOHO

In the West, this is the Traditional Usui Reiki. It has 3 levels of training (personal, practitioner, master, teacher) and 4 symbols.

TIBETAN REIKI

Developed by Ralph White using lineage to Tschen Li, who allegedly taught Mikao Usui. One level and 18, 19 or 25 symbols.

USUI/TIBETAN REIKI

Another version of Usui/Tibetan Reiki is taught by William Lee Rand. It has 4 levels and 6 symbols. Similar to Usui Shiyo Ryoho but levels one and two are taught together, and the 2 extra symbols are Tibetan.

JAPANESE REIKI TECHNIQUES

It has recently been discovered that there are differences between the Reiki that is used today and the original Reiki taught by Mikao Usui. New information and manuscripts have been found. For this reason, Japanese Reiki seeks to correct the difference by introducing original techniques. However, we may never know the exact original Usui Reiki Ryoho Gakkai.

The original methods include the 3 pillars (meditation, prayer, treatment) and approx. 30 techniques: using and chanting to help his students develop; massage as well as hands on healing; some group techniques; less formulated technique (timing and hand positions are intuitive rather than structured – This is called Byosen and Reiji Ho).

Mikao Usui also did not use symbols nor diagnose patients - the Reiki would just work on the person's energy. Mikao Usui taught that Reiki is a Japanese spiritual discipline and not a medical practice. Finally, Reiki had to be intended for the highest good of all.

EASTERN INFLUENCED REIKI

USUI REIKI RYOHO GAKKAI – Founded by Mikao Usui. 3 levels and Reiju. This is a sacred practice so is not open to everyone. The objective is spiritual growth and enlightenment. It is a society that was formed by Mikao Usui.

USUI REIKI RYOHO – Founded by Hiroshi Doi. 3 levels, 7 attunements, 4 symbols. Also uses Reiju.

TAIREDOU HEALING TECHNIQUE – Started in Japan by Morihei Tanaka, apparently at a similar time to Mikao Usui.

JOHREI – A religion from Japan that uses healing. Developed from Raku Rei. 3 levels, can be taught in 2 days. 4 non-traditional symbols. Uses same Master symbol as Mikao Usui and started a similar time to Mikao Usui.

VAJRA® REIKI - Founded by Wade Ryan in India. Comes from Johrei Reiki. 3 levels, 3 attunements and 4 symbols. Also meditation and mantra. Vajra is associated with Tantric Buddhism.

GENDAI REIKI HO – Founded by Hiroshi Doi, Japan to combine Usui with Western and Eastern Techniques. 4 levels and 4 symbols.

ICHI SEKAI REIKI – Founded by Andrea Mikana-Pinkham. 4 levels. Uses the first 3 traditional symbols and a Johre White Light symbol and a heart attunement.

IMARA REIKI - From Barton Wendell. One additional level for those who are already Usui Reiki Masters. No extra symbols. Meant to be a higher level to Reiki Master (Imara = "more").

JIKIDEN REIKI – Founded by Chiyoko and Tadao Yamaguchi. 4 levels, 3 symbols and 5 attunements. No Western influence.

JIN-KEI DO - From Ranga Premaratna. Mikao Usui's Eastern lineage (Hayashi, Tekeuchi, Venerable Seiji Takamori, Ranga J Premaratna). 3 levels of study and 4 levels of practice (Buddho EnerSense). 4

traditional symbols (except Cho Ku Rei different). Strong Indian and Tibetan Buddhist influences and focuses on compassion and wisdom (both of which make enlightenment).

JINLAP MAITRI REIKI - From the Tibetan Medicine Buddha and developed by Gary Jirauch. Is higher level for those who are Karuna Reiki Masters. Has 5 levels, 5 attunements and 25 symbols.

JINTAI-RAGIUM-GAKKAI – The Human Body Radium Society apparently created by Chiwake Matsumoto at a similar time to Mikao Usui.

KOMYO REIKI KAI – Founded by Hyakuten Inamoto, based on Hayashi. 4 levels and Japanese symbols and mantras. The purpose is spiritual growth and enlightenment.

MAHI KARI - A religion from Japan that uses healing. Uses same Master symbol as

Usui and started a similar time to Mikao Usui.

REIKI PLUS – Founded by David Jarrell. 5 levels. Developed from Usui Shiki Ryoho.

SHINNOUKYOU-SYOKUSHI-SHIKOU RYOHO – Violet Light Healing Method, used by Shinnoukyou-Honin religion in Japan at a similar time to when Mikao Usui was teaching.

REIDO REIKI – Founded by Fuminori Aoki. 7 levels with 5 symbols (one is extra "Koriki" symbol). Focuses on purification and self-growth.

REIKI-HO - Founded by Hiroshi Doi, Japan. 4 levels.

SATYA REIKI - From Japanese Eastern lineage. 3 levels (degrees) with 7 or 8 attunements. 4 symbols. Uses some of Barbara Ray's Radiance Technique and the Indian Chakra system.

TENOHIRA-RYOUCHI-KENKYUKAI SOCIETY - The Association for the Study of Palms, was apparently formed by Toshihiro Eguchi who broke away from Usui's original Usui Sensei healing group.

REIKI TUMMO – Founded by Irmansyah Effendi ("Grandmaster"). 3 levels. Claims to come from the Buddha and allows enlightenment in one lifetime.

USUI-DO - Created by Dave King and Melissa Riggall, in Japan. 13 levels. 4 symbols from Chinese Taoism / Buddhism. Traditional Japanese lineage.

ICHI SEKAI REIKI - Founded by Andrea Mikaha-Pinkham. Combines Usui and Johrei Reiki.

MEN CHHO REIKI OR MEDICINE DHARMA – Founded by Richard Blackwell (Lama Yeshe). It is based on Mikao Usui's notes. It has 3 levels. Uses Sacred Buddhist teachings.

BUDDHO-ENERSENCE - From Tibetan Buddhist Lamas such as Venerable Seiji Takamori.

ENERSENSE BUDDHA – Claimed to be from the Buddhist Lamas of Nepal, Tibet and Northern India. There are 4 levels.

WEI CHI TIBETAN REIKI – Founded by Thomas A Hensel and Kevin Rodd Emery (channeling Wei Chi). 6 levels with many hours of practice. Wei Chi said to be 5000 years old from Tibet. This is said to be the full version of Reiki.

WESTERN INFLUENCED REIKI (ADDITIONAL TECHNIQUES)

REIKI MARI-EL – Founded by Ethel Lombardi in 1983, one of Takata's students. She was an American healer of Reiki. Mari EL uses very gentle feminine energy, of Mother Mary. It is said to work at cellular level. As well as Usui Reiki, it uses Cranio Sacral Therapy and vibrational sound therapy, chelation techniques. It has 3 extra symbols. Advanced classes also available.

RAKU KEI - Created by Iris Ishikuro (one of Takata's original 22 Masters) and Cheri L Robertson, American Reiki Master Association. Iris Ishikuro was one of the first teachers to break away from Takata, by charging smaller fees for teaching. It has 4 levels and 7 symbols. Levels 1 and 2 are usually taught together.

RADIANCE TECHNIQUE® / AUTHENTIC REIKI® / REAL REIKI® – This is from 1986 by Dr. Barbara Weber Ray, who was taught by Takata in 1979. She is from America. This is "original" and "complete" Reiki passed to her through Takata, from the Usui lineage. However, she was the only one in the lineage taught the additional higher level Reiki attunements. After you have achieved Reiki Master (3rd level), you can receive symbols and be attuned for 4th, 5th, 6th and 7th degree Reiki.

REIKI (SEICHIM) – Seichim (pronounced say-keem) meaning "living light". It is thought to be one of the healing arts practised in ancient Egypt. It was rediscovered by Patrick Zeilger while visiting Egypt in 1980. 5 levels (facets). 8 attunements and 4 elemental rays: earth (Reiki), water, air and fire. Therefore, it claims to bring in slightly different energy to Reiki. There are variations of this: SKHM is Patrick Zellger's updated version of Seichim 1998; Sekhem is from Helen Belot 1991; Seichem is Kathleen Milner.

TERA MAI REIKI AND TERA MAI SEICHEM – Founded by Kathleen Milner in 1991. This was originally called Sai Baba Reiki. Tera Mai Seichem is another alternative to Usui Reiki – you have to redo levels 1 & 2. It was developed from Raku Kei, Usui and later on also incorporated Seichem. There are additional symbols though that were given to Kathleen Milner and Marcy Miller. These symbols represent extra elemental healing rays of fire (Sakara), water (Sophi-el) and air (two fold ray: Air and Angelic). Therefore, 4 new elemental healing rays and new symbols were introduced. There are 3 levels of learning (one, two, master) and each level has one attunement (i.e. 3). Students also take part in a water ceremony and Yod initiation.

REIKI (KARUNA) – Karuna Reiki was founded by William Lee Rand in 1994. 4 levels or just 2 levels if you are already a Reiki Master (Usui or William Rand Usui/Tibetan). 12 symbols. It has been developed from other forms of Reiki, such as Raku Kei, Usui and Tibetan.

Karuna is a sanskrit word used in Buddhism and Hinduism, meaning to release the suffering of others (samsara).

As we help others, we all benefit because we are all one, the same, one mind. It also uses meditation and chanting.

KARUNA KI - Karuna Ki was developed by Vincent Amador in 1999. It uses the same symbols as Karuna TM and Seichem Tera Mai Reiki TM but is not associated with either of those practices (although it has been developed from them). It is also the Way of Compassionate Energy to relieve the suffering of all sentient beings. 3 levels or just 1 level for Reiki Masters. There are 12 symbols but they have different meanings to Karuna Reiki. It is not trademarked – the idea being that it is open to all. It also uses meditation (toning) and chanting for spiritual growth and compassion.

LIGHTARIAN REIKI – Founded by Jeanine Marie Jelm in 1997 and is said to be from the Master Buddha and has 8 energy frequencies – Usui, Karuna, then

Lightarian. There are 4 training levels with 6 vibrations of energy (1st & 2nd; 3rd & 4th; 5th & 6th). There are no new symbols – just intention.

GOLDEN AGE REIKI – This has been developed from Maggie Larson (Shimara). It has 3 levels. It has some elements similar to Tera-Mai® with additional symbols.

SAKU REIKI - Developed by Eric Bott, German. 6 levels. Reiki with holistic therapy (herbs, nutrition, exercise etc). Combines Usui, Karuna and Tera Mai.

SOUL STAR SEICHEM – channeled by Terrance Blankenship in the winter of 2005. It has an extra master symbol, which can be used with Seichem or Usui Reiki. 1 attunement.

REIKI INFLUENCED FROM OTHER RELIGIONS

SUN LI CHUNG REIKI - From Yosef Sharon, Israel ("Grandmaster"). 5 levels and at least 6,400 symbols.

BRAHMA REIKI - Based upon shiva-shakti and began with Deepak Hardikar in India 1997. 3 levels and additional levels (Healing Through Balance and also Astral Travel levels).

SHAMBALLA REIKI – by John Armitage. Claimed to be used by St Germain in Atltantean healing times, who used 22 symbols. However, there are now 352 symbols (one for each energy frequency). 4 attunements and 4 levels.

ELOHIM REIKI – by Geomi in 2005. Elohim are the highest level of Angels. Must have done Usui Reiki Angelic Vajra and the Angelic Shakti to do this course. There are 12 symbols.

KUNDALINI REIKI – introduced by Mr. Ole Gabrielsen, a meditation master who channeled Master Kuthumi. No symbols, just intention. Lots of attunements.

GOLD REIKI – This is for Kundalini Reiki Masters. There are 3 levels and 3 attunements.

NEW LIFE REIKI - Founded by Dr V Sukumaran, India. 4 levels and approx 150 symbols.

NEW LIFE REIKI SEICHIM – Founded by Margot Deepa Slater (Reiki and Seichim Master). 7 levels, 36 symbols and 740 hours of training. Combines Tibetan, Chinese, Japanese and Egyptian.

CELTIC REIKI – By Martyn Pentecost. It uses Usui Reiki and the ancient wisdom of the Celts, such as the vibrations of the Earth and trees. It has symbols from Ogham, the sacred Druidic alphabet. 3 attunements.

CELTIC WISDOM REIKI – By Steve Malcolm and incorporates the Summer Solstice 2003. 10 Goddess symbols were channeled by Steve after a visit to Croft Moraig, Scotland. 1 attunement.

RAINBOW REIKI - Created by Walter Lubeck. It combines Usui Reiki with Angels, Shamanism, Feng Shui and Psychology. 3 levels with 8 attunements. 4 symbols for elements (air, water, earth, fire) and 5 animal symbols.

ELEMENTAL REIKI – by Rebecca Doolin. It uses symbols from Wiccan Goddess, Elemental and Paganism. 2 attunements.

ALCHEMIA REIKI – Founded by Reiki Master Kamala Renner and activates the fifth level.

ASCENSION REIKI - Founded by Alan Harris (Karuna Reiki) with Robert Nutt. Taught in 3 levels with 9 new symbols (7 chakra, 1 female, 1 male).

AMANOHUNA REIKI - Founded by Arthur Cataldo, Hawaii and has 10 levels (degrees).

AYURVEDIC REIKI – Created by Mohan Chute. It is based on Ayureda from the Vedic texts (from Lord Brahma), which is a holistic science for health. Disease is due to an imbalance of 3 elements of the body. The universe also has 5 elements, which are 5 types of energy. This Reiki training has 3 levels. You have to be Usui level 2 or Kundalini Reiki Master to do this course. No symbols.

BLUE STAR CELESTIAL ENERGY - From an ancient Egyptian school (via John Williams, South Africa 1995) but modified Gary Jirauch. It's achieved by channeling a spirit guide called Makuan and comes from an Ancient Eyptian Mystery School called Os-Mo-Ro-Pup. 14 symbols and 2 levels (7 Practitioner symbols, 7 Master). It is separate to Usui and Reiki. It's aim is spiritual growth.

PYRAMID REIKI – by Alaya. It uses Orgone energy. You must already be an Usui Reiki Master. There is a master pyramid matrix. There is 1 attunement.

LEMURIAN REIKI – This is a mixture of new energy and old energy from Lemurian times (said to be a lost civilization which existed in the time of Atlantis, near the Indian and Pacific Oceans).

GOLDEN ERA REIKI - This is Reiki linked to the lost city of Atlantis. It has one additional attunement and symbol. You must be Usui Reiki Master before you do this course.

DOLPHIN REIKI – by Mark Scott. It uses Dolphin energy (who are said to be Angels of the sea). 1 attunement.

MAHATMA REIKI – Leonie Owen-Rosenberg. 4 levels and 9 symbols. There are 352 levels back to the source or God. These method of Reiki aims for the highest possible source by using different Ascended Masters from different religions, as well as Angels and Archangels.

SACRED FLAMES REIKI (SFR) – by Allison Dahlhaus. Uses 7 Sacred Flames from 7 Chohans (ascended masters from different religions) and Archangels. There are no symbols, just visualizations and meditations. She says that all Reiki energies come from the same source – what matters is how we connect we them. 1 attunement.

SEVEN LEVEL – By Gary Samer, former Radiance Technique. 7 levels based on India Chakra system.

IMARA REIKI – This was channeled by Barton Wendel. It means "more" Reiki. It is on level 5 (the level "above" Karuna

Reiki) and mainly involves Angels, Archangels, Masters and Guides. 1 attunement.

CRYSTAL REIKI – by Malacti. Combines Reiki with crystals. 15 symbols.

REIKI USING ANGELS

ANGEL FLAMES REIKI – by Dr. Rev. Rebecca Meek-Horton. For anyone who is a master in Usui or Seichim Reiki. 3 attunements (can be done in one). One focuses on North, East, South and West. The second on a ball of flame. The third is for master/teacher level. After that, you can have 7 master attunements using the 7 archangels.

ANGEL REIKI – combines Reiki and Angels. There are 4 main Archangels used (one for each Usui symbol).

ANGELIC REIKI – by Kevin Core 1999. From St. Germaine, channeled through

Hari Daas Melchizedek (John Armitage). Combines Usui and Shamballa. Using Reiki symbols from Atlantean times and 30 Archangels. 4 levels (1 & 2, 3 & 4, Professional Practitioner, Master Teacher). 7 attunements

ANGELIC RAYKEY – by Reiki Master Sananda (channeling Archangel Michael). 3 levels. Uses traditional symbols.

ANGELS OF THE SILVER, GOLD AND VIOLET FLAME – by Anita Rushton. Re-founded by John Bride in 2010. Focuses on St. Germain and Archangel Zadkiel.

ARCHANGELIC SEICHIM – by Vincent Amador. It combines Seichim with Archangel energy. There are 12 Archangels for 12 symbols.

SAPPHIRES OF ANGELS REIKI – by Stephen Lovering. It is a follow on from his Colours of Angels course, but using Sapphire crystals (visually not literally) for each of the 7 main Archangels. 1 attunement with 7 empowerments.

OTHER HEALING

Spiritual Healing – This is not faith healing. Spiritual Healing is traditionally taught in Spiritual Churches, and is associated with their belief system (one God and spiritual hierarchy: Spirits, Spirit Guides, Angels, Ascended Masters from different religions e.g. Jesus, etc). There are different Spiritual Churches in the UK: The Healing Trust (formerly known as the National Federation of Spiritual Healers), Christian Spiritual Church, SNU Spiritualists National Union. Psychic development and Healing are kept separate. Healing is not for profit. Some organisations prefer "hands-off" (i.e. hovering rather touching).

Spiritual healing is usually taught over a period of approx. 18 months – 2 years. This includes a theory course, regular assessments and a patient log book. In addition, there is practical training for at least 30 hrs (Healing Pathway) or 100 weeks (SNU). The practical training sessions are supervised. The Healing Trust training is 4 courses over 2 years.

Some spiritual healers are cautious of other types of healing, such as Reiki, because correct use of healing takes a long time to learn and cannot be taught in 1 or 2 weekends. I agree and would recommend Reiki Shares to anyone learning Reiki, as well as the training courses and regular contact with a good teacher.

Angel Healing - Angel Healing is healing using Angels and Angelic frequencies. This is achieved through prayer and sometimes visualization without having had an attunement (e.g. Guardian Angels, Archangels).

There are also Angel Healing courses available with attunements and different levels of practice. For example, Diana Cooper School, Doreen Virtue ATP.

Distant Healing - All the healing types that I've listed above are hands on healing, face-to-face, but some of them also offer distance healing. Distance healing is where healing is sent to the person from another location. It should always be done with the person's permission and only for the highest good. It is used by e.g. Reiki level 2 and Master, Angel Healing, Spiritual Healing, Shaman.

Vortex Healing - This healing is thought to be from "Divine energy and consciousness" which dates back to Merlin (King Arthur). Merlin is one of the human teachers. It was rediscovered and developed in 1994 by Ric Weinman, when Merlin 'appeared' in his life. Ric is said to have had a transcendental experience, where he remembered being a Vortex Healer in his past two lives.

Faith Healing - This is healing that done through religious faith, prayers and rituals. It can be done at a distance or using face to face hands on healing. The emphasis is on God or the religious belief associated with the healing. Faith healing can also involve a pilgrimage to a religious shrine, such as Lourdes, France.

Shamanic Healing - Shaman are associated with different cultures and periods in history. Shaman communicate with the underworld (spirit world) using different techniques e.g. drumming, plants/herbs, rituals, meditation. Shaman do healing and medicine by working on the person at the 'soul level'. They have other roles such as earth healing, divination, shamanic journeying and soul retrieval. Typically, they will each specialise in a certain area of shamanic activity.

Old Testament – In 1 Kings Chapter 17 verses 7-24, the prophet Elijah healing the child of a widow with whom he was staying. Prophet Elisha uses a similar method in 2 Kings Chapter 4 verses 18-37.

New Testament – Jesus was a famous healer.

Jewish - The Jewish sect called the Essences, were also known as healers.

Cavemen – There is evidence of healing during the times of cavemen. Caves have been found with paintings on the wall that suggest healing took place.

Pagan times – Hands on healing was passed down in families in tribal and Pagan times. The old woman of the tribe was often its Priest, and it was her task to heal the sick.

It is also thought that Pagans taught a form of healing used by Jesus, based on the 4 elements and the 4 cardinal points after Christ's crucifixion.

Ancient Egypt - In Egyptian and Babylonia times, Priests used healing as part of the service available in temples of worship in Egypt, Greece and the Orient. By 1000BC the Egyptian, Imhotep became so famous as a healer that on his death he was deified as the Egyptian God of healing. Also, the Priest of Aesculapius.

Ancient Greece - Pythagoras, Hippocrates (460-377 BC) became a medical practitioner, and recognised how spiritual healing by the 'laying on of hands' alleviated some conditions, which was accompanied by a sensation of warmth and tingling. He described the energy healing 'as the heat that oozes out of the hands, being applied to the sick, is very salutary.'

Kings and Queens of France and Britain – When monarchs were held to rule by Divine right, it was believed that touching them with a coin and then wearing it was a cure for ailments. A `Touching Ceremony' first took place in the reign of Edward the Confessor and last in the reign of Queen Anne. The practice of 'royal healing' reached its peak at the end of the 17th century when Charles II was giving the 'royal touch' to around five thousand sufferers a year.

Chapter 4: Reikiself-Treatments

Please spend 3-5 minutes on the "basic positions"—more time on any area when necessary. In general, do a full body treatment one or more times per week (after your 21-day cleanse). Your in-between treatments can be 20 minutes total. When you need to conserve time, choose three positions you are most drawn to and stay with each area for five minutes. Your intention is always there to make the effects long-lasting. With practice, you will become very adept at honing in on what you are intending for yourself or others.

At the beginning of your treatments, create or use following Reiki blessings: Center and reverently bless yourself with a Reiki intention/prayer: **"Thank you Reiki for blessing and protecting me."**

"May I (and each body part) receive health, happiness, and wholeness today."

"I am youthful, strong, healthy, wealthy and wise. My body knows it and my body show it."

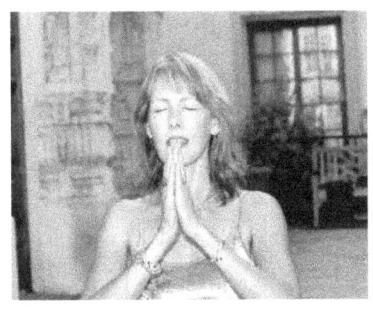

"Reiki within me. Reiki around me. Reiki to all I have contact with today."
"Thank you, Reiki, for this healing and blessings that come my way today."
Breathe for a moment, giving thanks for Reiki working with you and through you. You can create a short blessing to conclude:
Thank you Reiki for working in and

through me. May I continue to be blessed, healthy, happy and holy. Sat Nam.

Inhale to ground yourself. Stretch your arms and legs, toes pointed. You may touch your crown and "walk" your hands down your body for a deeper grounding. Drink plenty of water after you bless it with the Power symbol:

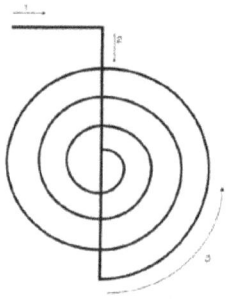

Be in gratitude for your life and all your forthcoming opportunities.

HAND POSITIONS AND BENEFITS

Note: Positions preceded with two asterisks (**) are considered "extra hand positions." You may include them in your regular self-treatments or when you are intuitively drawn to these areas.

Treating the Head Area

1: Eyes

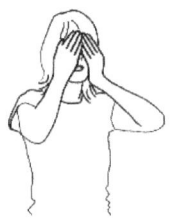

- Palms lightly over eyes
- Hands and fingers touching
- Base of hands over cheeks

Physical: Relieves eye strain, improves vision, clarity, balances pituitary and pineal glands, nose, sinuses, relieves headaches.

▱ Mental: Reduces stress, calms overactive mind, relieves anxiety. Improves clarity, focus, concentration, mental energy. Aids decision making and confidence. Addresses, "What am I not willing to look at?"

▱ Spiritual: Awakens third-eye point, intuition and inner wisdom.
**2:Eyes/Temples

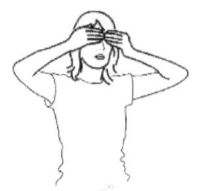

▱ Fingers over brow point
▱ Hands cupped around temples
▱ Saturn (middle) and Sun (ring) finger tips touching

▱ Physical: Eyes: Vision, clarity, pituitary and pineal glands. Balances right and left sides of the brain. Relieves stress and headaches. Improves memory.

Mental and Spiritual: Benefits are the same as position #1.

3: Ears and Temple Area

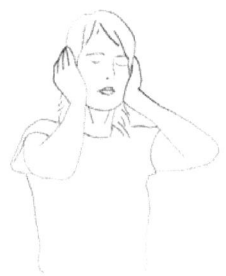

Palms over ears and temple area
Fingers together pointing up

Physical: Balances right and left sides of the brain. Relieves tension from jaw muscles, migraine headaches, improves memory, ear problems, seizures, shock, motion sickness. Boosts hormonal responses.

⬜ Mental: Stabilizes emotions, reduces worry and depression, creates new ways of thinking and being, balances male and female aspects, calmness. "What am I not willing to hear? What am I not listening to?"

⬜ Spiritual: Left ear relates to inner voice, right ear to outside guidance from a material perspective.

4: Crown

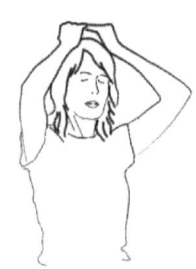

⬜ Hands on top of head
⬜ Fingers touching
⬜ Palms close to top of ears

▫ Physical: Balances the left and right brains, pituitary and pineal glands. Releases endorphins. Provides relief to pain, seizures, shock and motion sickness.

▫ Mental: Relieves worry, hysteria, stress and depression; promotes serenity and dream recall. Increases creativity, calmness, memory enhancement.

▫ Spiritual: Openness and Oneness with the Universe.

5: Base of Skull/Center of Head

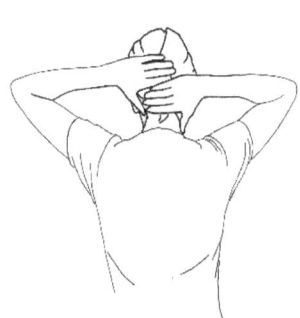

▫ Upper hand at head center
▫ Bottom hand over neck base/occipital

bone

◫ Thumbs pointing down at side of neck

◫ Physical: Balances cerebellum, medulla and nervous system, weight, spine, pain relief, speech problems, sleep cycles. Energizes brain and provides more oxygen in the hemoglobin.

◫ Mental: Relieves fear, worry and depression. Helps to accept and release past difficulties and long-term memory enhancement.

◫ Spiritual: Protects the psychic gateway from psychic attack. Promotes openness and universal vision.

**6: Lower Face

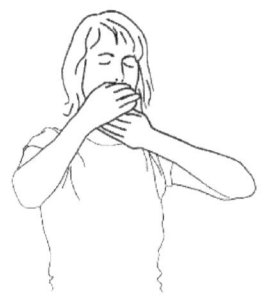

- One hand cupped over mouth
- Other hand over jaw and chin
- Physical: Helps mouth, gums, teeth, jaw line, TMJ. Balances blood pressure. Releases tension.
- Mental: Mouth represents need for nourishment. Teeth problems represent procrastination.
- Spiritual: Nourishing yourself from the soul level.

Treating the Front Area of the Body

7: Neck and Throat

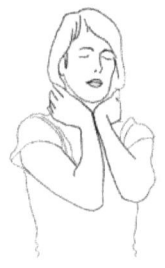

⬜⬜ Base of palms and wrists touch throat
⬜⬜ Fingers gently wrap around neck

⬜⬜Physical: Regulates active/underactive thyroid and parathyroid glands (aids postmenopausal women), lymphatic system, metabolism. Balances blood pressure (carotid artery). Affects larynx, throat, tonsils.

⬜⬜Mental: Reduces suppressed thoughts and emotions. Relieves anger, hostility, frustration. Improves confidence, self-esteem and ability to communicate with honesty. Creates a clear mind and well being.

☐ Spiritual: Truth and creatively expressing. Creating from the power of word and feeling.
8: Lower Throat and Upper Chest

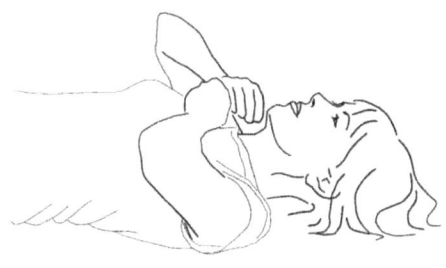

☐ One hand over "high heart," thumb relaxed

☐ Place other hand over throat/on top of other hand

☐ Physical: Provides extra boost to throat center, high heart, thymus gland, immune system, circulation.

☐ Mental: Communicating with

compassion, kindness and joy.
☐ Spiritual: Freely creating, expressing, and living Divine qualities of love, joy and bliss.
☐ Repeat: "I am bountiful, blissful, beautiful."

9A:HeartCenter

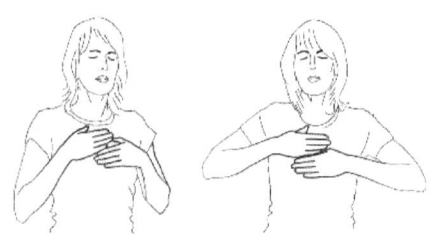

☐ Hands crossed, angled or horizontal over lungs/heart
☐ Finger tips touch if in horizontal position
☐ Physical: Balances heart, thymus gland, immune system and circulation
☐ Mental: Giving, receiving and accepting love and nurturance with compassion, kindness

and joy.
 Spiritual: Freely creating, expressing, and living Divine qualities of love, joy and bliss.
 Repeat: "I am bountiful, blissful, and beautiful."

**9B: Breasts
 Cup each one in your hand.
 Milk Glands: For mastitis, place hands under arm, against side of upper chest. Place one hand in each armpit.

 Mental: Breasts represent mothering and nurturing. The left is for spiritual nurturing and the right for material needs. Breast problems generally represent a refusal to nourish the self—you put others first or are over motherly and overprotective.

10:SolaPlexus

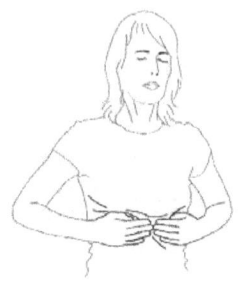

◫ Palms at bottom of ribcage/over solar plexus

◫ Saturn (middle) fingers touch

◫ Physical: Balances liver, spleen, gallbladder, pancreas, nervous system, diabetes, stomach and digestion.

◫ Mental: Releases fears, chronic complaining, anger, grief, diversions and being overwhelmed. Improves personal power, self-determination, clarity and focus.

◫ Spiritual: Receiving peace that passeth all understanding. Receiving higher energies.

11: Navel

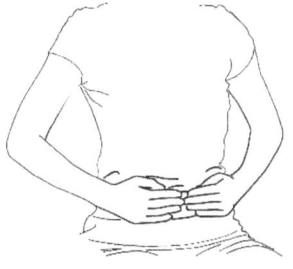

▥ Hands one inch below or on navel
▥ Saturn (middle) fingers touching

▥ Physical: Balances small intestines, transverse colon, upper ascending and descending colon, lower liver, pancreas, gall bladder, spleen, bladder, sexual health.

▥ Mental: Releases fear, aggression, anxiety, depression, manipulation and control. Balances sexual feelings, obsession, repulsion and assimilation of new ideas.

☐Spiritual: Promotes inner power, worthiness and strength.

**12:HipBones

☐ Cup palms on hip bones
☐ Fingertips angled towards groin

☐Physical and Mental: Balances hip area. Heals varicose veins and leg pain. Eliminates emotions stemming from sexual issues.

13:Groin

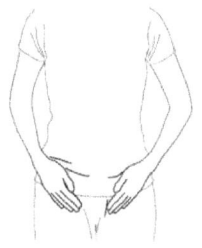

⃞ Slide hands down and form a V
⃞ Fingertips are over pubic bone

⃞ Physical: Improves lymphatic and urinary system, blood and neural circulation to legs, intestines, lower part of ascending and descending colon, appendix, rectum, prostrate, ovaries, uterus, bladder, constipation, diarrhea, hips, migraines. Prevents ovarian cysts and uterine fibroids.

⃞ Mental: Increases energy, vitality, abundant living, stability, security, flexibility and creativity. Helps balance sexual issues stored in cellular memory.

☐ Spiritual: Expansion of higher awareness. Deeper connection to Mother Earth.

Treating the Leg and Feet Areas

**14: Mid-Thigh

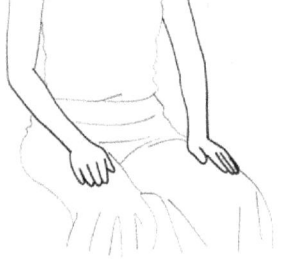

☐ Palms slide down to middle of thighs
15A: Knees

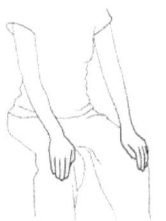

■ Hands cupped over each knee
■ Physical: Thighs, knees, shins, ankles and soles of feet. Relieves leg cramps, varicose veins and circulation in legs.
■ Mental: Knees represent humility and being able to bow down to authority figures.

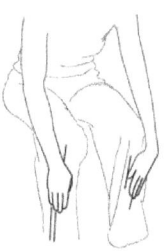

**15B: Shins: Place hands over shins
16:Feet

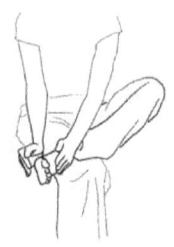

- One hand over front of foot
- Other hand on the sole
- Switch feet and repeat
- **Alternate:** Each hand on top of each foot, then switch to place one hand on each sole.
- Ankles: Represent the foundation of self and being flexible.
- Feet: Represent your life direction. "Where am I heading?"
- Toes: Represent the minor details in life.

Treating Arms and Hands
Extra Arm Positions

These are extra positions to use for a wellness boost or when feeling any discomfort in the forearm area to the fingers.

**17: Elbows

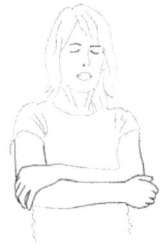

▢ Hands hold elbows
▢ Physical: Benefits tennis elbow, arthritis
▢ Mental: Elbows— elbowing your way through life. "Get out of my way! I need some space!"

**18: Wrists
Physical: Improves carpal tunnel and loosens wrist tension.

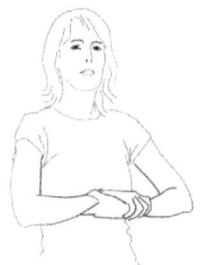

19: Fingers (Not Shown)
⊞ Same arm postures as wrists
⊞ Slide hands to cover fingers
Mental: Being flexible in the way we handle things.
Hands: Balancing being a giver and receiver.
Fingers: Represent the minor details in life.

Back Positions

⊞Upper: Carrying your burdens and those of others
⊞Middle: Emotional area and old issues
⊞Lower: A need for perfection; financial and security issues

20:Shoulders

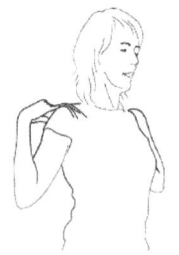 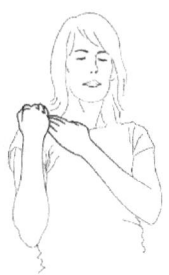

Depending on your arm flexibility and comfort levels, there are a few variations:
- Right hand on right shoulder
- Left hand crosses to right shoulder
- Do same for left shoulder

Or:
- Arms bent, fingertips on shoulders
- Right arm bent with palm and fingers on top-right shoulder
- Left arm bent with palm and fingers on top-left shoulder

🔲Physical: Shoulders, lower neck, heart and lungs, upper spine, neck injuries. Reduces bursitis, upper lung and lymphatic congestion and tension in neck.

🔲Mental: Releases heavy emotional and mental burdens (left side one's own, right side of others), past issues. Instills calmness and centering.

🔲Spiritual: Ability to receive higher energies, communication, serenity, flexibility.

21:UpperBack

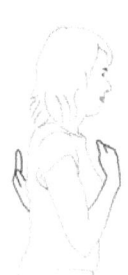

☐ Right hand over upper chest
☐ Left arm reaching around to upper back
☐ Left hand at base of right shoulder blade
☐ Switch hands to other side

☐ Physical: Shoulders, heart and lungs, upper spine, neck injuries. Reduces upper lung and lymphatic congestion.

☐ Mental: Releases heavy emotional and mental burdens. Instills calmness and centering.

☐ Spiritual: Ability to receive higher energies, communication, serenity, love and compassion.

22: Mid-Back

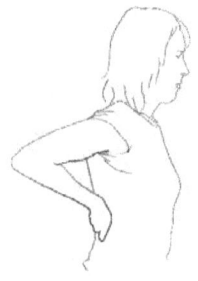

⊞ Left and right hands touching lower back ribs
⊞ Middle fingertips touch

⊞Physical: Energizes lower lungs, heart and thymus gland, pancreas, stomach, spleen, mid-spine, kidneys, adrenals and solar plexus. Healthy adrenals support function of kidneys, bones, bone marrow, and spine.

⊞Mental: Alleviates control issues. Assists with trust issues and deep relaxation.

23: Small of Back/Lower Back

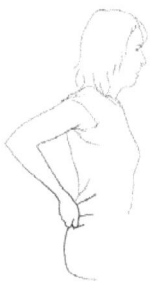

▫ Hands on lower back, forming a V with fingers pointed down.
▫ Physical: Relieves lower back problems. Reduces stress.
▫ Mental: Improves expression of suppressed emotions. Promotes feelings of worthiness and joy.

24: Coccyx/Base of Spine

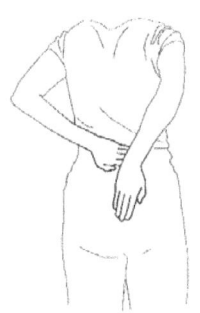

⊞ Form a letter T
⊞ Left palm horizontal
☐ Right palm vertical over tailbone

⊞Physical: Relieves discomfort in lower back/sacrum, hemorrhoids and hips. Balances reproductive system, rectum, small intestine and colon.

⊞Mental: Old patterns released to allow new behaviors. Increases mental power and quick creative thought reflexes.

25:     Sit   Bones/Roots

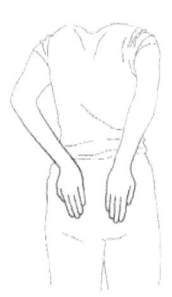

⊞ One palm over each buttock.
⊞Physical: Relieves discomfort in sciatic

nerve. ❏❏Mental: Relieves instability and financial worries.

Chapter 5: The History Of Angels

Synopsis

The word angels is derived from the Greek word angelos, which means messenger.

The origin of angels in history is rather complicated to figure out, due to angels or like spirit beings being found inside many cultures around the Earth.

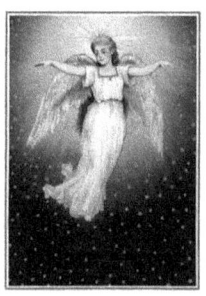

Angle History

Angels are found inside 3 key religions: Judaism, Christianity and Islam. Yet, angels, or divine people who help others, were likewise found inside Sumerian, Babylonian, Persian, Egyptian and Greek writings, too.

While perhaps called different names, benevolent spirit beings rather similar to angels may likewise be found inside additional religions, mythologies, and lore.

Today, a lot of individuals believe in demons and that they're fallen angels. This teaching originated in the Hebrew text of Isaiah about Lucifer getting cast out of heaven with a third of the angels following him to the Earth.

A common description occasionally given of angels is that they're "beings of light," which are occasionally described as "frightening to behold" due to their tall height, purity, and sheer might. A few will likewise describe angels as having wings and perhaps even halos. Yet, the western notion of wings and halos developed through ancient religions and mythology.

Images of angels looking like humans, but with wings, were an ancient idea that exemplified benevolent spirit beings as arriving from a "higher place" or the "heavens." Wings were a simple way to express the idea of angels moving back and forth (or even up and down) from the spirit world to Earth and then back once more. A lot of ancient gods were frequently depicted as birds or as bearing wings (think Egyptian, for instance). By the fourth century (AD), angels were broadly seen as having wings inside western cultures, while wings were nearly non-existent inside the Eastern faiths.

A lot of ancient civilizations had placed wings on their deities, creatures and champions, so it was natural for Christian artists to look to pagan civilizations for inspiration. Christian artisans were prompted to add wings to angels by viewing Greek art. Muslim artists looked to Persian versions as their inspiration for wings upon angels. During this same time, Christian painters likewise adopted the idea of the halo from the Greeks and Romans who had utilized them previously.

But, a lot of times in the bible, angels seem to be men and are described as such from Genesis (e.g. when Jacob wrestles an angel) to Revelation (e.g. the letters to each of the churches are addressed to the pastors, or angels of every church). Even the name supplied to the archangel Gabriel means, "Man of God." Moreover, Jesus was attributed as teaching (in Matthew) that in the resurrection, those raised would be "as" (or like) the angels of God in heaven. This statement is additionally clarified by the similar text written in Luke 20 which says, "for they (the raised) are angelic."

Today, a lot of individuals look to angels for help or even intervention during crisis. A general modern-day description of angels is discovered in a lot of stories of helpful, but mysterious strangers. These stories frequently tell of an individual who seems to come to an individual during a time of need, supplying a word or help of some sort, then mysteriously vanishing fast. During these experiences, the messenger or helper is indiscernible as an angel, however seems as a loving, caring human. Similarly, spirits who come to soothe and lead dying individuals through the transition from this Earth unto the light (heaven, promised land, and so forth), are frequently described as angels, however are occasionally discovered to be deceased loved ones or friends of the one about to pass on.

Therefore, angels appear to have a really close association with human beings, perhaps even closer than we may think, when one analyzes biblical descriptions along with accounts of personal experiences. Summarizing angels described inside religion and inside personal experiences in general, we know they're benevolent spirit beings that bring messages, assisting mankind; angels appear in human form; and angels have been described specifically as the spirits of human beings inside the spirit realm. Maybe the term angels is a word to universally describe bodiless, yet enlightened spirits of individuals, who help other humans on both sides of the grave.

Chapter 6: The Benefits Of Reiki

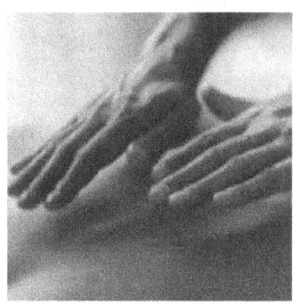

Reiki can balance the body at any level. If you are tired, you can get a Reiki treatment to feel rejuvenated and refreshed. If you are anxious, you will calm down and relax. If you are stressed out, you will feel comforted. If you feel overwhelmed, you will learn to take some time to think through your emotions and your thoughts. Whatever you feel, getting a Reiki treatment can be very helpful. A lot of people see and feel the difference immediately after the first treatment and if you repeatedly get treatments, you will see the benefits grow and last.

There are a lot of excellent benefits that Reiki can provide. Although it is a very simple process, it is able to produce wonderful and profound effects. Aside from healing the body and making it less vulnerable to diseases and illnesses, Reiki also aims to promote the health and positivity of the mind and body so you can enjoy your life better.

You have to be aware, though, that Reiki is not a miraculous cure that can instantly eliminate your disease. Certain conditions that have long been in the body cannot be cured with just a few Reiki sessions. In order for the Reiki to assist in your recovery, you have to want to recover and become active in your healing process. You might need to make some changes in your lifestyle and remove the aspects in your life that cause you stress and negative emotions.

Reiki supports your overall well-being and health. Reiki treatment is safe and will never interfere with any medical treatment that you might be receiving. Reiki can be performed on patients in the operating room, patients who are undergoing chemotherapy or patients who are pregnant. If you are required to take prescription medications, Reiki can support those medications and make them work better. Reiki is very effective and can be performed on anyone, regardless of age, level of health, ethnicity, religion or background. Reiki helps people improve themselves and provides them with a greater sense of meaning in life. Reiki treatment can successfully balance the body's systems, which can help make them better able to cope and handle various health conditions including:

Cancer

Heart diseases

Anxiety

Depression

Chronic pain

Infertility

Neurodegenerative disorders

ADD or ADHD

Autism or developmental delays

HIV or AIDS

Crohn's disease

Irritable Bowel Syndrome

Traumatic brain injury

Emotional illness

Fatigue syndromes

End-of-life care and bereavement

Migraines

Asthma

Skin conditions

Flu or colds

Ulcers

Arthritis

Back problems

Low self-esteem

Poor self-confidence

Reiki treatment works directly on restoring the body's balance on all levels and works on the root of the problem instead of just relieving symptoms or masking it. The good thing about it is that there is no need to have a certain condition to get the benefits. Even if you do not need to treat something, you can still get a Reiki treatment.

There is no need for you to wait until you get sick to get a Reiki treatment. You can get a Reiki treatment whenever you want, but if you are confused and are wondering when you can have one, it can be performed when:

You are sick but simply want a relaxing and therapeutic treatment.

You feel down or sluggish and need a boost to increase your energy levels.

You are on medication.

You feel pain.

You are undergoing surgery or stressful treatments like chemotherapy.

You are stressed out.

You are tired.

You are pregnant.

Reiki is for everyone and can be performed anytime you want. It not only can heal adults, but can also heal children, babies, the elderly and even your pets.

Chapter 7: The Principles Of Reiki

It is expedient that Reiki practitioners remain in alignment and not live any contrary to the greatest force that controls the universe and to that effect are guiding principles. They are five in number, referred to as Gokai—very profound, and must be rightly understood and stuck to the heart. The principles are the very foundation of the Reiki philosophy as regards the practitioner's personal life code and not some harsh or restraining rules, laws, or boundaries, and as such, no one is expected to adhere to them. With it, every Reiki believer's balance and perspective is shaped aright.

They are more like spiritual guideline which offer you the chance at self-introspection and allow you to work on yourself each day absent a sense of guilt or pressure.

For your personal good and general benefit, these cardinal Reiki principles—keys that help build the system's foundation—are better interpreted as a mean to expand your outlook and actions. In order to rid the planet of all forms of ills, and ultimately promotes serenity and coordination, a measure of purposeful determination is needed. That is why it's good to apply these principles daily so you can open yourself up to the Universal Life Force that resides already in your being as well. Discrepancies exist in the practice of Reiki and the wordings of the five cardinal principles may reveal it but it doesn't mean they are different in what they communicate essentially.

These cardinal Reiki principles may sound absolutely simple that you would think sticking by them through the entirety of your time is a possibility, but it isn't that way at all. The world we currently live in, so incongruent in many ways, makes it so.

It doesn't, in any way significant, reflect and reinforce the principle. A life permanently opposite it is what many people exhibit, but as for those that live by them, they experience more harmony in their life. These principles are the driver, and anchor of the Reiki practitioner's mindset.

Each principle starts with the word "Today." The reason for this is because is because the Reiki idea believes that what creates and dictates the future is this present moment, not yesterday, not tomorrow. By living the principle it allows you to deal with this moment, forgive yourself and those that did not in the previous moment. Focusing on "today" as regards the cardinal Reiki principles gives you the prospect to be able to fine-tune your conduct and actions in such a way that you can start being in perfect alignment with the principles even if your way of life has been contrary before.

Your way with them towards personal profiting and to the benefit of others is something exclusively up to you. You can let them thrive as the subjects of your meditation sessions. You can turn them to affirmations and say them loud to yourself. You can also write the 5 cardinal Reiki principles down or carry them as muses everywhere in the recesses of your mind. It's yours to use as it suits and there is definitely no wrong way to implement them into aspects of your life as they aren't one-way traffic. If you uphold them and live to its creed, they will serve you well in your self-improvement journey.

Don't be in any way disheartened if you find the Reiki principles difficult at first because with enough sheer will and frequent practices it will soon become effortless. Soon enough you will begin to notice a great improvement in your personal life and the influence your new being can have on others.

Principle 1

"Just for today, I will not worry"

What is the foremost font of negative energy in the world today if not stress? And what causes stress and deep-seated anxiety if not worry? When you worry, you tend towards a state where imbalances readily permeate your mind, spirit, and body. You stand at risk of a mental degradation and your whole being gives you away as unpleasant and unhealthy. When you are under the sway of stress, there is a way you get taken as though you are uncouth, mad, and impatient. And guess what, this creates further imbalances and concord between your body, mind, and spirit.

You can really part with stress if you stay with the habit of viewing each obstacle in your life as an opportunity. Learn to approach situations with a positive attitude and you can easily alleviate stress.

When you sneak this first principle into your life and it becomes a driving force within your soul, it will make you realize that all the precious time you have in this world can't just be spent on worrying as the eventual stress isn't worth it. To stay calm and approach each day with beams of hope and gratitude lacing your face is a more worthy vocation.

See, if you really must live a life of serenity—a life filled with fun, this principle is a necessity. It is only a matter of time if you start to follow it as it will lift your overall mood, and ultimately your performance in life.

Principle 2

"Just for today, I will not be angry."

You can take my word for it when I boldly declare that the second will fall seamlessly into place if you can effectively incorporate the first Reiki principle into your life. Anger is an emotion that rides on the wings of stress. Sometimes, a standalone emotion gets the better of us as humans and like boulders across the neck weights us down. We get our liberation when we start to learn how to control our concerns and untold worries. We get better by responding to people, not just reacting and that is a really giant forward step. When we understand what triggered our anger, we are a step closer to mastering the act of regaining our emotional outbursts.

There is nothing unnatural in having feelings that border on jealousy, envy, among others. Nobody should slate you for you and you shouldn't be hard on yourself either because you are perfectly normal and functioning well and in no way are you a bad person for feeling that way. The big problem is when you allow them to grow so bold and strong in your heart that they spread a blanket of shade which impedes your natural love and light and smears your spirits.

Principle 3

"Just for today, I will do my work honestly"

It is kind of straightforward to quickly conclude this principle as revolving around corruption—something like calling in sick when you are not or making sure that you mastered the dark arts of adding zeros to financial digits.

It is far more than that.

Out of the five cardinal Reiki principles, this is the one that borders not just on honesty, but on integrity—personal integrity you might say. Maybe you often procrastinate or even slack at your work? Maybe you are versed at exaggerating your progress? Perhaps you are one who has become addicted to taking a few extra minutes more then you should during breaks?

Just for "today", decide to focus, function, and deliver at your peak. Be honest with yourself and those life has placed around you. Unleash yourself and hold nothing back because doing otherwise amounts to cheating others.

Principle 4

"Just for today, I will give thanks for my many blessings"

If you are given to the attitude of gratitude, you become healthier, kinder, and happier, says many scientific research sources. If we learn to wield the power of gratitude—probably the most important gift we can give as humans—we will go on to live a more fulfilled life. Learn to talk a halt on regular basis, pause and acknowledge the many blessings that have flooded your way. Right now, many of them are there but you may not see them because you have trained your heart to acknowledge only scarcity-what you do not have. Think about it: you are very much alive, have a fully-functioning body, a roof over your head, and can draw in barrels of oxygen per day.

It isn't just about the material things—things easily grasped by the scope of your sight, hearing, and touch. Appreciate the nice weather you've got as a cloak around you. Say thanks for having for having good sleep and waking up to full light daily, say thanks. Nothing improves our lives exponentially as when we come to the realization that blessings are everywhere. Why not start a gratitude journal today and see how effective and resounding your life will become by implementing this principle in your everyday life.

Principle 5

"Just for today, I will be kind to my neighbor and every living thing"

When we allow positive thoughts to permeate our hearts, we end up creating a serene atmosphere that causes a blossoming of more positive thoughts which eventually bring more things to feel positive about in our lives. It is the same when we do otherwise—negative experiences streaming from negative thoughts. It's quite a great feeling to know that we did something that brought immense feelings of betterment, be it in mood, feelings, or experience, to another. When you do something for someone next time, pay keen attention to how they change. It's something that will spur you in to do even more as it is a very empowering experience.

Practicing these cardinal principles is a simple way to improve virtually every area of your life and put it on an upward pedestal. It is something that requires only some measure of commitment—not laborious efforts—and you can actually start right away. There is guaranteed positive changes that will come upon your life if you can strive to live within the framework of these powerful Reiki principles.

Chapter 8: Reiki And Buddhism

Reiki is intimately linked to Buddhism and when you do your Reiki I, you might want to explore Buddhism and its beliefs and principles. Buddhism is one of the very few religions that has never promoted violence to impose its views. As a matter of fact, not only that, but Buddhists are actually not that interested in converting people. They don't even consider Buddhism as a religion but more as a philosophy. It is interesting to know that in some Buddhist countries, Christianity and Buddhism exist hand in hand in the practice of many people. They are both Christians and Buddhists.

The story of Buddha is quite extraordinary in itself. He was a married and soon to be a King. He decided to leave everything behind to look for peace and find a relief from suffering. There is a wonderful book called **Siddharta by Herman Hesse** that I recommend, if you want to read about the Buddha's life. This might lead you to want to learn more. What is essential to understand is that Reiki is the way of healing that was practiced by the Buddha. So the link is very intimate. This does not mean that Jesus' healing was not as powerful. In fact, some say he went to India and learnt a lot of his teachings from Buddhists. Reiki was practiced for many years by monks only and kept a secret from the masses. Reiki is a sacred practice that needs to be treated with respect.

Buddhism has for centuries made the link between the mind, the emotions and the body. Modern psychology recently discovered what Buddhism has taught for centuries. Buddhism is a holistic approach and as such is very beneficial for students of reiki to deepen their knowledge of human nature but also of illness and wellbeing. It is important to understand that reiki does bring the consciousness to the part of the self that is creating the illness, to understand it, but also focuses on the part of us that is healthy, peaceful and divine. It aims at reconciling the two and by rebalancing these polarities; it can create harmony, which is the basis for health.

Buddhists believe in reincarnation. Many things have been written on reincarnation and karma and a lot of misunderstandings have been spread. Karma is the law of action. It means that for every action there is a reaction. It does not mean, as it has often been perpetuated that if you hurt someone, then you will be hurt in the same way in return. I see the law of karma more as a necessary learning curve and to be given the opportunity to make amends and to learn by ones' mistakes. This means that if you understand and become responsible for your thoughts, words and acts – and all three rank equally as important – then you will progress on the law of karma, sometimes without having to go through the experience of being on the receiving end of your own doings. This also means, as far as I am concerned, that I can detach from wanting to know if someone is going to be "punished" or has made amends for how they hurt me, because the law of karma will take care of it. It is out of my hands. I don't need to interfere. I don't need to judge. I find it very liberating. It opens the way for true unconditional love. You can then just see people's actions as mistakes that will lead to learning for them. And of course, this applies to us.

Reincarnation is a wonderful concept because it liberates us from the pressure of perfection. I believe, and this has been documented, that most of the main religions used to include reincarnation as part of their teachings but carved it out when religions started being used to control the masses. The effect was to rob the person of his or her direct link to God, which was then given to the Priest, Rabbi, Imam, and to instil fear of sins. This enabled religions to rule and govern people in the most intimate details of their lives. Reincarnation on the contrary, leads to theories that you actually plan your life for certain lessons with the help of a council of wise light beings. There is thus no justice or injustice in your lot, as you are unfolding a plan that enables you, if you choose to learn the lessons and transcend the situation, to progress as a human being. Progression is to become more loving, more accepting and more giving. Unfortunately, we often have to learn through hardships. Even thought you plan your life in advance, you still have free will to conduct it as you please. And that's where humans mess things up and that's ok too. A lot is due to the fact that we have much clearer vision of what we want to achieve before we come to this earth and once we get here, we forget everything and get caught up in the drama. Our guardian angels know that and they never get angry or impatient with us. They know we will get there in the end.

Buddhists practice awareness, something that us westerners have forgotten a long time ago. The miracle of mindfulness is simply the shift that happens to us when we live totally in the present moment and keep our peace regardless of circumstances. We are not here talking about extremes. Let's take the example of a meal. How often do you take the time to bring your awareness to the sensations in your mouth whilst you chew your food? Do you even take the time to taste it and take notice of the change in the texture and taste as your saliva starts to digest it in your mouth? Mindfulness is the practice that also leads to meditation and the quieting of the mind.

This leads me to mentioning how important it is to practice meditation if we want to be potent channels for the reiki energy.

Chapter 9: The Importance Of Initiation Size

Reiki is an approach to utilize the vitality in your grasp to adjust and revive the existence power vitality inside us. At the point when our life power vitality is high, we are less inclined to become ill. Numerous individuals who have been sick have profited by physical, mental and passionate recuperating from this hands-on vitality treatment. Through Reiki attunements, you can figure out how to take advantage of the existence power vitality and renew and mend yourself as well as other people. For some, the attunement or commencement procedure begins in 1stDegree Reiki Practitioners Healing Training. For other people, it is the formal commencement into mending others performed at the Reiki ace level.

This book examines the job of attunement in Levels 1, 2 and Masters Reiki preparing.

With numerous reports in the media about vitality mending, more individuals are interested and looking for an introduction to vitality recuperating. Standard Reiki attunements is a demonstrated method to guarantee long haul great health. It has come to notice that one of the attractions of Reiki is that anybody can figure out how to utilize it. Reiki bosses mend by widespread vitality, or Qi, that is gone through the palms. This life-renewing vitality practice is passed on from ace to student.

Reiki doesn't just treat physical wellbeing yet in addition enthusiastic, mental and otherworldly health. Ensuring your life power vitality is adjusted is the most ideal approach to guarantee all encompassing wellbeing. This Japanese recuperating strategy is progressively being utilized close by Western prescription as a component of the mending process. Thus, request is expanding for prepared experts who can perform Reiki attunements.

Solution to choosing Reiki Initiation Master

Picking the privilege Reiki ace is essential to the achievement of your attunements in every one of the three degrees of training. Since Mikao Usui created Reiki in 1922, numerous varieties have pursued. Request that your planned educator clarify their preparation and experience utilizing Reiki. Ask her to discuss her way of thinking of Reiki and bow it might contrast from that of other Reiki masters. And critically, get some information about any progressions or upgrades to her Reiki program from the customary practice.

The International Center for Reiki, for instance, underlines the convention of the customary Tibetan methods just as the

Usui Reiki techniques. This program professes to make changes in accordance with the first Reiki technique. Truth be told, there are a few ancestries of Reiki instructed in Japan today – some of the hidden and others vigorously impacted by the Western procedures. Guarantee you comprehend the Reiki procedure being offered. Specifically inquire as to why this framework is the best for you.

Functional contemplations incorporate booking. When is the class held and for how long? Weekend courses have turned out to be well known however would a weeklong retreat be better for you? Charges shift extraordinarily today among schools. To direct Reiki to other people, every one of the three levels are required. At the ace level, you will be started into recuperating others. Consider at the time, cash and different assets you will require to finish Masters level Reiki.

Reiki is more physically private than many specialist understanding relationships. Ask yourself how agreeable you would lie on a table for an hour getting Reiki medications from your educator. Reiki includes opening yourself up profoundly and emotionally. If you wind up inclination guarded or bashful, keep on talking Reiki teachers. Assess your mood. Do feel upbeat around this person? Does the educator make you like yourself?

Planning for the Attunement Process

Clear your calendar of all commitments. If you have a ton of work and family worry during your Reiki class, it will be more earnestly to open yourself up to the vitality procedure. Try not to design any significant get-togethers during your Reiki commencement forms, particularly those including liquor.

Sanitize your arrangement of poisons. Take out caffeine, liquor, meat and sugar from your diet. Consider fasting for a couple of days.

Think for an hour every day. This is a significant advance that will enable you to quiet your psyche and manage your vitality stream before the exercises start. You will get more from Reiki preparing on the off chance that you are now raising your vitality vibrations.

Attempt and maintain a strategic distance from unpleasant circumstances and individuals. Once more, this is to help guarantee a quiet, thoughtful attitude.

Invest more energy among nature. Another unwinding strategy. Stroll to take a shot at a bright day. Take a walk around the recreation center or by the sea as opposed to staring at the TV.

The Reiki Attunement Process

What is Reiki Initiation?

Ace Usui got his capacity to take advantage of Reiki vitality through an otherworldly reflection. The custom of passing Reiki down from ace to understudy proceeds. Attunement is another and later term for Initiation, or reiju in Japanese. Pamela Miles, a Reiki specialist, makes a noteworthy distinction between the terms attunement and inception in her blog. Understanding the genuine significance of inception will extend your Reiki practice. Quickly, attunement is frequently characterized as the strict exchange of all inclusive vitality from ace to understudy, supplying the understudy with the capacity to turn into a healer. Though inception alludes to the start of learning a training. Learning, as Miles notes, includes posing inquiries, and learning can be constant. Like the nonstop renewal of vitality, the professional ought to constantly build up their abilities as a vitality healer. While inception better catches the genuine plan of Reiki recuperating, we will keep on utilizing the famous term attunement here. Yet rather than consider attunement a privilege of entry as a vitality healer, attempt and think about every attunement procedure as the start of a constant learning process.

Reiki Attunement Through the Three Reiki Levels

The attunement or commencement procedure happens in every one of the three degrees of Reiki: Reiki 1, Reiki 2, and Master level. At each level the Master starts the understudy with more grounded mending vitality as the understudy moves to more elevated amounts of vitality vibration.

Reiki 1 includes four commencements of the physical body. To become an affirmed level 1 Reiki expert, you will find out about the vitality heights of the body, the Reiki hand positions, and Reiki life systems; and at last how to utilize the Reiki vitality framework to recuperate yourself as well as other people. When this learning is effectively aced, the Level 1 Reiki attunement must be given by a Certified Reiki Master. The function more often than not takes 20 or 30 minutes.

Reiki 2 starts the unpretentious or air body. Three Reiki images are educated – control, mental and separation. Notwithstanding the sacrosanct symbols, 2ndDegree Certified Reiki Practitioners Training teaches extra images and hand positions. A few courses will likewise show removed Reiki recuperating at this stage.

The Reiki Master level starts the understudy into instructing Reiki. The Master image is educated. A few Masters allude to this third organize as the official attunement or inception arrange as a vitality healer. At Level 3, you will figure out how to do Reiki attunement on others.

Separation Reiki Attunement

Numerous individuals offer the chance to get Reiki and different types of vitality mending a good ways off. While some separation healers have demonstrated that they draw from an amazing vitality source, most Reiki experts don't prescribe separation mending. Episodically, a large number of those utilizing separation recuperating report that the vitality isn't as solid. A few bosses accept that the physical touch is basic to convey the required mending vitality. Handy contemplations incorporate challenges getting neighborhood references and joining nearby Reiki gatherings to whom your healer likewise has a place. In the case of preparing in Reiki or looking for mending, similar capabilities for picking a Reiki ace ought to be utilized.

The Reiki Ideals

Learning the Reiki procedures and going through all phases of attunement/inception is just piece of the way toward turning into a mindful vitality healer. You should likewise maintain the good and moral norms of a Reiki vitality healer. The Reiki Ideals were created by Reiki organizer Usui Mikao. The Reiki Ideals guarantee the sound and dependable routine with regards to Reiki. They are an attestation that you are the healer and in charge of your own demonstrations of mending. The first Reiki beliefs are as per the following:

· The mystery specialty of welcoming bliss

· The marvelous medication everything being equal

· Only for now, don't outrage

· Try not to stress and be loaded up with appreciation

· Dedicate yourself to your work. Be thoughtful to individuals.

· Each morning and night, join your hands in petition.

· Ask these words to your heart

· furthermore, serenade these words with your mouth

Check out Usui Reiki Treatment for the improvement of body and psyche

When you have learned Reiki, the capacity to mend yourself as well as other people physically, rationally, sincerely and profoundly is with you for a lifetime. Like any learning, on the off chance that you seek after nonstop learning – that is, continually addressing and finding out more – your Reiki mending vitality will stay solid and all the more profoundly receptive to the general vitality source. While recuperating others is a steady wellspring of reconnection with the vitality source, getting attunements now and again from different bosses will keep you finely sensitive to the vitality source.

Inception or attunement?

Some time after the demise of Hawayo Takata* in December 1980, "attunement" firing springing up. Numerous Reiki experts presently use it only for the procedure Mrs. Takata alluded to as inception (reiju in Japanese).

Despite the fact that the inception procedure is baffling, "commencement" is entirely clear. It alludes to starting.

Inception is the procedure by which an ace offers with an understudy the capacity to rehearse. Commencement ancestry keeps training alive and is regular in profound Asian customs.

The procedure of inception is innately baffling; what it achieves — empowering us to rehearse — isn't.

Similarly, as the pith of training is to start once more, commencement can be rehashed. Usui offered reiju to his students each time they assembled to rehearse.

The ascent of "attunement" appears to have put a conclusion to addressing. It urged specialists to see Reiki as a specific vibration of "vitality" to which individuals should be "adjusted" so as to rehearse. This disarray — that one is receptive to vitality as opposed to started into training — has taken on its very own existence and is currently for the most part introduced as certainty.

In any case, it is anything but a reality. It's a conviction. What's more, if Reiki practice is predicated on conviction, it's never again a training; it turns into a religion.

When you take a gander at it that way — which is how individuals outside the New Age people group will, in general, take a gander at it — is it so astonishing that some religious society is against Reiki practice?

Demystifying inception, in a manner of speaking

It's difficult to demystify inception because the procedure itself is supernatural. In any case, while the inception procedure is baffling, what it achieves is down to earth and normally unmistakable. Individuals who get a Reiki inception might see something during the procedure of commencement. However I would say they see the impact.

As a youthful Reiki ace, I committed the error. Maybe all new aces make: I blabbered.

After some time I came to welcome that my activity isn't to clarify Reiki. Or maybe, my duty as a Reiki ace is to show understudies how to rehearse Reiki, to move them to rehearse day by day self-treatment, and to give them the certainty that they really can rehearse effectively.

Is inception enough?

I realize every one of my understudies needs are the inceptions; I likewise realize they don't have the foggiest idea about that. I can't anticipate that they should trust me, nor do I need them to. I need understudies to build up their very own certainty. What's more, nothing I state can make certain the path in-class practice does.

In my First degree classes, we move into the first of four inceptions offered in Hawayo Takata's genealogy directly after the welcome and presentations. I at that point lead the understudies through their first altered Reiki self-practice. After this short introductory practice, and before they open their eyes, I request that they see any little contrast between the manner in which they feel currently contrasted with how they felt when they began.

When I've delicately driven them out of their training session, the understudies share what they saw during their first practice. I don't recall the last time somebody didn't see anything.

In any event, individuals feel more settled, increasingly focused, progressively loose — and that is not how they expected to feel sitting discreetly in a gathering of outsiders.

The procedure of commencement is innately secretive; what it achieves — empowering us to rehearse — isn't.

Reiki Initiations are here to push you to reconnect with your picked life way and to turn into a channel for this Universal Life Healing Energy. It is the establishment for your own healing in your consistent life and a chance to pass it onto other living creatures in the hour of this major vivacious progress from the third dimensional Energy to the fifth dimensional energy. It is a mending practice and a method for living with profound regard, sympathy and empathy for the Soul and each living being including yourself, other individuals, creatures, plants and Mother Earth.

Reiki Initiations can raise your cognizance to a more prominent level and bring understanding of your actual way and subsequently the motivation to your own picked educational experience, the significance (or certainty) of disease or a problem, and learning involved. Through Reiki Initiations your own vitality is being raised, your levels of awareness and mindfulness start developing – so significant as of now of transformation, to stay aware of this approaching high fifth dimensional Energy.

SO DO WE NEED INITIATION TO BE ABLE TO USE REIKI?

Indeed, we should be started by a Reiki Master Teacher, who has been adjusted accurately themselves. Reiki is a high, sacred Life Healing Energy and to have the option to arrive at that level our energy and awareness should be raised. We can not do this by itself, a Reiki Master should be there for us to take us however those stages. This is the way Master Usui started his understudies. It is a significant minute in each person't life when we believe we are reconnecting with our actual self and the Holy Source that individuals call Mother/Father God.

In contrast to other recuperating expressions, Reiki is passed from ace to understudy through a Reiki attunement that allows the understudy to interface with the all-inclusive Reiki source. However, the attunement enables you to turn into a vessel of Reiki, and move Reiki vitality for yourself as well as other people. So while you can find out about Reiki in a book and learn hand positions, until you have been receptive to channel Reiki, you can't really rehearse Reiki.

So, what is Involved for Each Reiki Attunement?

Be aware that in a Reiki level 1 attunement, students are receptive to three unique images, each speaking to an alternate part of Reiki vitality: control, mental/passionate equalization, and separation recuperating. Every understudy gets attunements to these three images, four separate occasions, and with every reiteration the association develops.

Therefore, the attunements for Reiki level 2 and Reiki ace are comparative, yet include various images, each with alternate importance to opening your vivacious pathways.

So, what Does It Feel Like to Get an Attunement?

Getting a Reiki attunement is a profound ground-breaking experience, as your lively pathways are opened by a Reiki ace. This vivacious opening permits the Reiki vitality to stream uninhibitedly through your body to affect your wellbeing and the soundness of others.

The sentiment of a Reiki attunement is an individual one, yet understudies regularly report that they feel a helping of their body and shivering from their head to their toes as the Reiki vitality pathways are opened.

The opening of an attunement has the impact of enhancing other lively mending and directing pathways, and understudies report that accepting an attunement causes expanded instinctive mindfulness, and improves any intrinsic clairvoyant affectability.

How Do You Prepare for an Attunement?

Meanwhile, how you get ready for a Reiki attunement relies upon your very own profound practice. Opening a vigorous pathway is no light issue, and keeping in mind that it's not carefully important to do anything so as to get ready to get a Reiki attunement, most understudies decide to reconnect with their own otherworldly practice before their attunement, to increase the general impacts of the attunement and amplify its transformative power.

One prescribed arrangement for planning for a Reiki attunement involves a 3-day rinse before your attunement. Abstain from eating overwhelming nourishments, limit or dispose of caffeine, sugar, tobacco or liquor. Invest your energy perusing or pondering instead of sitting in front of the TV. Endeavor to discharge negative feelings, for example, outrage or desire.

These arrangements will enable you to be increasingly prepared to acknowledge the otherworldly change and urge the attunement to have significant, long haul impacts on your life and prosperity.

Does an Attunement Need to be Renewed?

When you have been sensitive to Reiki, the Reiki vitality will course through you for an incredible remainder. Your capacity to channel and move Reiki vitality stays with you, as the endowment of Reiki tails you and encourages you for an incredible remainder.

So what Are the Benefits of Receiving Attunements Remotely?

In-person classes are regularly instructed rapidly, absent much time for understudies to consolidate the data. The attunements are given as once huge mob toward the part of the arrangement, without time for the understudies to plan for the significant otherworldly change that an attunement involves. By studying remotely, you can learn and incorporate the advantages of Reiki at your own pace, and take a couple of days to set yourself up for your attunement before you get it.

Reiki is an enthusiastic practice, and a great part of the Reiki you get and convey all through a mind-blowing remainder will be a ways off. Starting your Reiki venture remotely encourages you get ready for an existence of Reiki without outskirts.

Chapter 10: Daily Reiki Practice

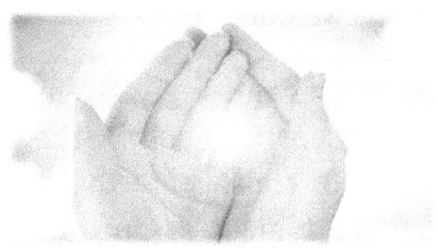

By Ananya Sen

Hello everyone! This is one of those articles that I am guided to write about. Most of the articles I write are inspiration I receive during meditation, but sometimes the universe or the guides tell me what to write about. This is not my personal opinion. It's guidance.

And I have noticed they often ask me to write about topics that are generally questioned by practitioners. So here goes, what do you Reiki practitioners do on a daily basis. What can you do for daily practice in the various levels of Reiki that you're attuned to? Why aren't you MEDITATING?

1. **First Degree Practitioners –** yes you must do self healing and chakra clearing or chakra balancing. You can also try a little bit of meditation, making a Reiki ball between your hands and sending it to people and situations.

You need to activate Reiki everyday because you have just been promoted from the normal vibration to a higher vibration. The energy needs to align with your chakras and body systems.

2. Second Degree Practitioners – self-healing – yes either directly on yourself or via distance, but you have to heal yourselves at this degree. The jump from the first to the second degree is high, so your vibrations are suddenly raised and you need to keep up.

Now, I always insist on meditation. There is no better option to raise your vibration, increase your healing ability and connection with the divine. You can start with five minutes per day, do open eyed meditation with one or more of the Reiki symbols. If you want to align with your higher self I suggest you do meditation with HSZSN. The guides tell me that there's no point in coming to Reiki, if you're going to be a lazy practitioner!

3. Third Degree / Masters & Teachers – I hope you meditate on a daily basis, because for you guys it is soul level healing. You are on your way to enlightenment, which is what the ultimate purpose is of the soul. If you're not meditating, start now! At this level, you will begin to experience ascension or enlightenment symptoms and it is going to be uncomfortable. Neuralgia, body ache, sleeplessness, dry mouth, depression, pressure on the crown chakra etc are some of the common symptoms of the ascension process.

To be able to deal with this and to be constantly connected with the source, please meditate on the Master symbol. It will basically do everything for you. If you feel your third degree energies are low, then build your rapport with the master symbol. It will align you completely to the high vibrations of the third degree.

Note for Everyone - Meditation is the key to become more spiritual, increase your healing power and even increase your income / business or whatever it is that you do. Meditation opens the third eye, which is the seat of intuition and intention. Reiki is about intention. If your third eye is weak, your intention becomes weak and your energy flow will be weak as well. Thank you for listening.

Shortcut to Self-Healing

By Sunetra Dasgupta

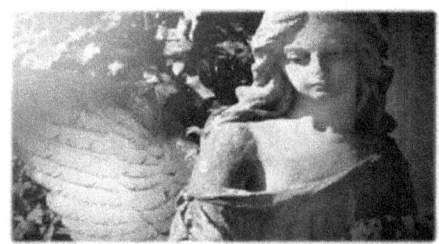

When I was first introduced to Reiki... how excited was I! It was on my mind from the moment I woke up till the time I went to bed. I kept on reading a lot about Reiki and its practical uses to enhance my practice. My Reiki teacher, who is also my sister, told me continuously: "Do Reiki and Be Reiki."

I was ever ready with the energy to heal and help others but I was bored while doing Self Healing. Even though I know how important it is, Self healing made me yawn like there is no tomorrow.

My sister shared with me a beautiful method of self-healing and amplifying our Reiki.

The method was to connect with any God/Archangels/Ascended Masters everyday for 10 -15 minutes and send Reiki to them. I have broken down the steps for everyone's benefit.

Method:

1. Sit in a comfortable place where no one is going to disturb you, put on some healing music and connect with the distance healing symbol to any God / Archangel / Ascended Master. You may connect mentally or keep a photo.

2. Send Reiki for 10- 15 minutes. Talk to them during this time. This is important. Ask them to clear your Aura & chakras for Self healing.

3. Ask them to amplify your Reiki Power, make your connection stronger with them, or simply ask for blessings and guidance on any issue. They really like to listen to us!

In my experience, this method has worked for me in many wonderful ways. They do listen to us and show us the right path in such a subtle way that we do not even come to know there has been a divine intervention.

They also shield us from negative and psychic attacks. I have also requested them to be my "Reiki Bank". Which means whenever I feel the need to increase the heat in my hands, I ask them to give me some of their energy. For instance I may say: "Dear Buddha, please send me some of your energy to increase my Reiki flow!"

You can practice this as often as you can. It is good to pick one Ascended Master / God / Angel for a week or so. The results are incredible! Not only has this made me a better practitioner, but also made me understand the spiritual aspects of Reiki.

10 Ways to Use Reiki in Everyday Life

By Angie Webster

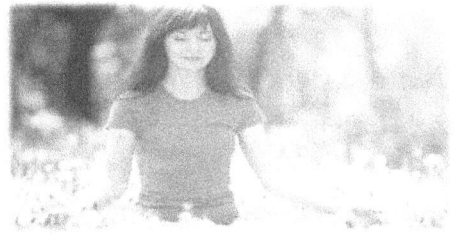

Reiki is not just something I practice on myself to stay well or on others to assist them in their well-being. Reiki is an integral part of my life. It is something I acknowledge throughout my day, from the moment I wake up until I fall asleep at night. I see it as a vast and living energy that connects me, in a very real way that I can feel, to my Higher Power. I ask the Reiki energy to assist me, for the greatest and highest good, in most everything I do throughout my day. I understand it as a critical part of my spiritual path.

Here are some ways you can incorporate Reiki into your day. Use your creativity to see what other ways you can think of to invite this beautiful energy into your life.

1. Infuse your intentions and prayers for the day with Reiki when you first wake up. Also consider doing self Reiki for a few minutes first thing in the morning.

2. Send Reiki to your food as you make breakfast (or any meal) and also bless it as you sit down to eat the meal. You can send Reiki to your groceries when you harvest them from the garden or buy them at the store as well.

3. Meditation is a wonderful time to tune in to the Reiki energy, allowing yourself to become more familiar with it or to allow the energy to flow to yourself for self healing.

4. When you leave for the day, take a moment to send Reiki to your car and to the trip ahead. You can also send Reiki to the destination you are headed to and to any situation you will be arriving into.

5. Incorporate Reiki into any spiritual practices you have throughout the day, contemplating ways that this life force energy surrounds and interconnects us all. Think of how this understanding might affect your spiritual practices of compassion, kindness, forgiveness and gratitude.

6. Most animals very much enjoy Reiki! It is often preferred from a distance, though your own pets may love it hands on. You can also treat their food, water, bedding and toys with Reiki.

7. If you have houseplants, cut flowers or a garden, honor and nourish them as they honor you. Give them an energy exchange by offering them Reiki! It is also useful to treat their soil and water with Reiki.

8. Use Reiki to cleanse and protect the energy of your home or work environment. Reiki chi balls are very useful for this. You can also use Reiki to quickly clear and charge your crystals.

9. If you are having a difficult time or a conflict in a relationship, you can send Reiki to the situation and to yourself to help ease the difficult emotions and bring about a resolution to the issue.

10. At the end of the day, you can send Reiki to your final prayers and to your sleep, asking that you be shown the resolution to any issues you are struggling with as you sleep.

Remember the Reiki precepts each day and practice using Reiki in as many ways as you can think of and you will soon find that it becomes a part of you. Your spiritual practice and Reiki will be intertwined and your life will be a spiritual practice. That doesn't mean you will be perfect, but you will see how to honor life and yourself in more ways all the time.

Chapter 11: How To Practise Reiki After Attunement

Hand Positions Illustrations

Practising Reiki every day is compulsory. One has to practice minimum of **3 minutes** per point. No need to worry if time exceeds more than III minutes per point, but practising less than 3 minutes per point is not welcome.

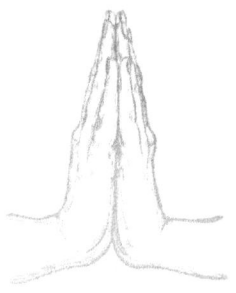

Do Namaskara

Say thanks to Reiki

Thanks to all Reiki Masters

Thank yourself

Now start practising hand positions, cover the area approximately with the palms of your hands. Complete the cycle of 26 points in a day. For best results do all the points in a single stretch it approximately takes 1 hour 30 minutes.

One can practice Reiki any number of times a day. Sit in a quiet place and practice Reiki don't chant any mantras or listen to any kind of music or watch TV. Observe variations of warmness in your palms or in the particular part where you are practising Reiki. Observe changes in yourself before and after practising Reiki. As you practice Reiki, observe and spend more time on parts which "draw more energy" compared to the other parts. If you don't feel difference in the energy

flow yet, don't worry; just spend equal

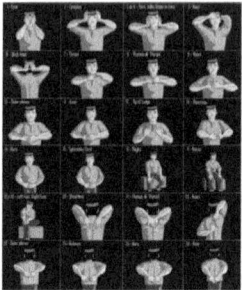

time on each position.

Our breathing pattern indicates our mental status and harmony, proper breathing is very important for a healthy life. We need to change our breathing pattern to clear any mental, physical or emotional problems. Many meditations are based on science of breathing, even Reiki focuses on breathing.

Once you start practising Reiki, it automatically changes your breathing pattern according to the requirement of healing-energy to a particular organ/problem. As you change the hand positions while practising Reiki, you can notice changes in your breathing pattern automatically without any effort. As well as you can feel the difference of warmth and energy flow in different parts of your body.

After initiation some may experience symptoms of physical and emotional detoxification, as the Reiki energy works on both emotional and physical blockages.

Physically some people may catch up with fever, body aches, dysentery or may over sleep. The body flushes out the toxins at first. On emotional level they may feel quite exhausting at times, as it removes long standing fears, unwanted anger, stress, tension and frustrations.

Reiki energy blends well with any form of healing. It increases positive effect on all forms of illness and negative conditions like headache, stomach ache, surgery, cold, stress, anxiety, heart disease, cancer etc. It even reduces the side effects of medical treatments like chemotherapy; it helps to reduce the time needed to stay in the hospital post-operation or delivery by increasing body's natural ability to heal itself.

One can practice Reiki any number of times in a day and at any time of the day. Reiki works at night too. No need to worry about particular place, time, food habits, etc.

Your life will change positively once you start practising Reiki regularly. To achieve peace, happiness, good health and mindset just practice Reiki! Practice Reiki! Practice Reiki! That's all you have to do.

Develop the habit of practising Reiki for yourself before you fall asleep at night and when you wake up in the morning. Reiki is like regeneration; it cleanses your mind, body and spirit.

Chapter 12: Introducing You To Beginner Yoga Exercises

There are some basic yoga exercises that you can do to get you aware of how yoga works. One of the best of these routines is the sunlight salute. This is what I use in the mornings to awaken the body and soul at the same time. If you do this in an inspiring place, when you are more experienced at yoga, you really will find that it's helpful in making you more motivated, in helping your body to avoid cramps and aches and pains, and that it sets the mood into positive mode to greet the day.

The sun salutation is first rate for helping you to get the breathing exercises in time with the movements.

Sun Salutation

For this yoga position, you can start by standing on your yoga mat, with your feet shoulder width apart. Your back should be straight and if you can lift the chest area a little, this gives you a great breathing position. Place your arms by your side. Inhale and relax and then exhale and bring your palms together in front of you. Keep your hands in this position for a few moments. Instead of being a closed prayer position, separate your fingers and continue to breathe in and out being conscious that you are breathing correctly as explained in the breathing chapter.

Inhale and move the arms down by your sides. Exhale and move your arms outward and upward so that they are stretched above your head. Remember that the breathing is everything. Exhale and draw your body forward moving your arms out to the sides like a swan. If you need to bend your legs then you are permitted to do this. Remember, you are a beginner and this isn't about hurting yourself.

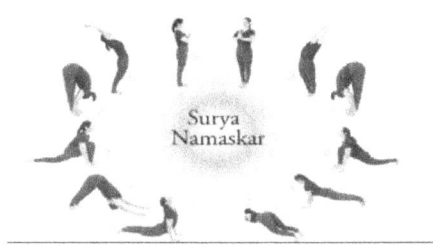

You can see all of the movements of the sun salute in this image and you need to follow them. So far we have explained as far as between number 2 and 3 and you are on your way to touching your feet. Pull one leg back as shown in the image, followed by the other, but remember to breathe with each movement. If you follow the sequence shown all the way through, you end up in the same position where you started and that is the whole intention of this exercise.

The sunlight salute is something that you can practice because it introduces many other positions such as the downward facing dog, etc. and also makes you go through a series of exercises which touch each group of muscles in the body and that's a great work out for the beginning of your yoga session. If you go over each of these movements again and hold each movement for a moment, you are learning more positions than you may imagine, so that the sequence makes a perfect routine for a beginner of exercises that play a part in yoga practice. They are by no means the only exercises and we have added more in the following chapter that you can practice and become proficient at and that help certain parts of the body or certain problems that you may have with mobility.

Breathe – move – breathe

Chapter 13: Living Without Worry

In this chapter, I want to look at the second Reiki principle "Just for today, do not worry".

Whereas anger is an emotional response, worry is a thought process. Did you know that you have over 60,000 thoughts per day?! I'd love to know who actually got paid to count them!

To understand worry, we need to understand how we think. Thoughts help us to make sense of the world around us. The brain receives information and manipulates it into a model in the mind which we then perceive as thoughts.

Thoughts

These thoughts can be positive or negative in nature.

Your thoughts carry energy vibrations – and before you think "Oh no here she goes again with all that mumbo-jumbo energy vibe thing", science backs this up!

Scientists can measure thoughts in the brain using specialised equipment and they have shown that thoughts do indeed have specific vibrations, and furthermore, there is a difference between positive and negative thoughts.

Positive ones have higher vibrations as we would expect.

The new world of Quantum Physics is highlighting that we are all connected energetically and that the universe as we know it is actually all energy and created by the observer: -

A fundamental conclusion of the new physics also acknowledges that the observer creates the reality. As observers, we are personally involved with the creation of our own reality. Physicists are being forced to admit that the universe is a "mental" construction. Pioneering physicist Sir James Jeans wrote: "The stream of knowledge is heading toward a non-mechanical reality; the universe begins to look more like a great thought than like a great machine. Mind no longer appears to be an accidental intruder into the realm of matter, we ought rather hail it as the creator and governor of the realm of matter.

(R. C. Henry, "The Mental Universe"; Nature 436:29, 2005)

Fascinating stuff – we actually create our own reality. Your thoughts are things and they matter! You get what you focus on – the Law of Attraction is real!

You know this – if you have pessimistic thoughts, for example "I'm going to fail this test – I am no good at this subject" or "I can't do this right at all – it's going to be a terrible day", more often than not you will prove yourself right. You will fail the test or have a bad day and then you will use that experience to self-prove your theory. You will say, "See! I told you I couldn't do it"!

Usui was really on to something when he said, "Just for today, do not worry". It is so much deeper than simply not worrying – it really means to look at the state of your thoughts and focus on a more positive thinking pattern.

It is time to become aware of your monkey mind - your internal dialogue.

How do you talk to yourself?

Are you aware of your thought patterns at all or is it all just background noise?

When I was thinking about this subject and this chapter I thought about getting into the brain and explaining how it works.

I then thought about talking about the higher self, the conscious self and the subconscious, in an effort to explain the thinking process to you.

I decided against all that – quite simply Reiki is simpler than that. It is not about how the brain works or how you think. It is about shining the light of awareness into your thinking patterns so you can make an informed choice about how to perceive the world around you.

Just like having an angry emotional outburst is a choice you make, so is the act of worrying.

Born worrier?

You may perhaps believe that you are a born worrier. Is that true? As a baby did you worry? Did you come out of the womb worried? No, of course you didn't. Babies don't worry – it is a learned behaviour.

Your behaviour, thought patterns and beliefs are all programmed from an early age from the people around you and from your environment. If your parents were worriers, then you will most likely inherit a similar pattern.

If you were constantly told "Money doesn't grow on trees" or "You have to work hard and pay the bills" then you will believe that money is difficult to come by and that working hard for a living is the only way to get money. This is an example of a limiting belief.

How you view the world will be based on your belief system but the good news is that you can change that!

If you are already a naturally positive thinker then great! If not, then you may need some help to address your thinking patterns.

Penelope Quest, in her book "Living the Reiki Way" discusses the concept of Faulty Thinking. Here are some of the examples she gives: -

● Black & White thinking – seeing things in a polarised way with no consideration for middle ground

● Blaming – not taking any responsibility for disappointments or let downs, preferring to blame others

● Comparing – comparing yourself less favourably to other people

● Filtering – you filter out the positives and only hear the negatives

● Jumping to conclusions – automatically assuming the worst or negatively making assumptions

● Labelling – you have uncomplimentary labels for yourself or others

- Mind reading – you think you know what other people are thinking based on your own ideas

These are just some of the things which can be listed as "Faulty Thinking". This type of thinking creates or contributes to upsetting emotional responses such as anger, guilt, anxiety and poor self-esteem.

I am sure you can find something in that list that you are prone to do – I know I can!

The secret to living without worry is to begin to control the monkey mind and to look at the perspective you have.

Perspective

Perspective is like a window – which window do you look out of?

Perhaps your window is clouded with judgement and pessimism so that when you look through it all you can see is more of the same. Or perhaps your window is sparkling and clean making everything you see clean and fresh.

I read a story on social media recently about a young married couple who had just moved into their new home.

Each day the lady across the road would hang out her washing on the line and the newly-wed girl would comment to herself "Oh my goodness – look at the state of her washing. She really doesn't know how to get her clothes properly clean!"

She even remarked to her husband about the state of the neighbour's washing. As the days passed she couldn't believe that her neighbour would hang out such dirty laundry.

One day she was amazed to see that the laundry was beautifully clean and she ran to tell her husband that the neighbour had finally managed to get her washing properly done.

Her husband just smiled and said "No darling, I simply washed our windows."

So you see the newly-wed girl had been making judgements and assumptions because she was looking through a dirty window.

Which window do you look through each day?

A useful tool to identify your internal dialogue is to write down how you describe yourself. In this exercise it is OK to write completely honestly and put down both positive and negative traits – only you will see this so don't censor yourself.

Write down a description of yourself – if it is easier, write it in the 3rd person as if you are talking about someone else but make it true – exactly how you would describe yourself.

Once you have done this then place a tick beside all the positive words you have used and a cross against the negative ones.

Count up your scores – are you more positive than negative or vice versa or are you pretty balanced?

Now score out all the negative things – this is an exercise in positivity!

Replace them with their opposite meaning and make them positive instead!

This is just a quick way to identify how you think – whether you are an optimistic (glass half full) or pessimistic (glass half empty) thinker. Maybe you are a realist – the glass can be refilled! The point is to identify your thought patterns.

Worry is essentially fear – the fear of failure or the fear of the unknown.

It lies in a "What If?" mentality. Worrying doesn't actually achieve anything. Think about a time when you worried about something – did it make any difference to the outcome of the event? Of course it didn't.

Worry does nothing except steal your peace of mind and keeps you awake at night.

You should not bury your worries – that is not what Usui was advocating when he said "Do not worry". It is perfectly normal and human to have concerns and worries – Usui was suggesting that you do not let these things preoccupy you entirely.

Shine the light on the thing that worries you. Ask for help if needed or choose to let go of the need to control how things will work out. None of us know the future and nobody can control it so worrying about it will not help in any way.

As with the emotional responses we looked at last time, notice where you feel the anxiety and worry in your body. Breathe into this area and if Reiki attuned then give Reiki to the situation to help you calm down.

If it is a forthcoming event, for example, a driving test that you are worried about you can use visualisation techniques to help you feel better. Close your eyes and see yourself in the situation, coping well. See yourself driving confidently and with no problems. See the examiner giving you a smile and congratulating you on passing the test.

The human brain cannot tell the difference between a real event and a vividly imagined one – which is why scary movies are so good at raising your heart rate!

Using visualisation techniques is a tried and trusted method, so when you next feel worried why not give it a try?

I have an inner sanctuary that I go to in my mind when I feel worried. It is my safe place - my happy place. It gets used frequently and in particular when I am at the dentist!

Dealing with worry

Essentially there are two ways to deal with fear (worry) – you can either change what you think or change what you do. The choice is ultimately yours but here are a few more things you can try: -

Smile! It is hard to worry with a smile on your face.

In Amy Cuddy's book Presence, she points out that psychology follows physiology. In other words your body language will impact your body's reactions.

She talks about power posing – for example – standing with your hands on your hips and deep breathing while visualising yourself as strong and confident.

In studies where people did this, their stress hormones lowered significantly and their testosterone levels increased – making them actually feel (and behave) more confidently.

So try it – smile and notice your body. Unclench your teeth and lower your shoulders and take a few deep breaths – this naturally helps to relax you and the worry starts to fade.

I would also suggest exercise and fresh air.

Getting outside into nature really helps with grounding the fear and moving it into a more positive emotion. Exercising releases endorphins which are the body's natural feel good drugs.

Move your body – put on some music, dance, laugh and smile.

If worries are significant or getting you down then talk them over with a friend or counsellor. Seek help if you need it. Don't feel afraid of reaching out for help.

I hope this has helped in some way to help you live without worry. Reiki is a journey of self-discovery and Usui gave these tools to help us navigate the way.

Remember the concept of "Just for today ..." and if worries get the better of you one day then you can simply start again the next day and set the intention "Just for today I release worry".

Chapter 14: Supreme Preceptor

15.1. A New Era

We live in this world of intense competition and advanced scientific facilities, with a mental depression that was born out of fatigue and distress unable to cope with the constantly changing trends. This is the reason why people wholeheartedly reach out for any new spiritual exercise that promises a way out for them. Unlike perception of olden times, the new age masters clad in ultra-modern attires, are amongst the most popular. But the new age that has brought with it new thoughts, faith and theories is not designed for adoption of joy by everyone. But a natural way of life amidst natural surroundings that proves conducive for the intake of electro-magnetic rays is sure to guide us to lost kingdom of God within us.

15.2. Cosmic Energy – Preceptor

This cosmic energy therapy should be learnt from a competent preceptor, which depends largely on your luck and good time. As saint poetess Avvaiyaar observed:

"Pandu Munaippadhu Arisiye Aanaalum Vindu Umi Poanaal Mulaiyaadhaam-konda Paer Aabal Udaiyaarkkum Aagadhu Alavindhi Eattra Karamun Seyal"

"Even powerful persons cannot accomplish any task undertaken singlehandedly. Just like the rice, though equipped to generate by itself, cannot do so if it is stripped of its outer shell, similarly a preceptor's guidance is an absolute necessity for success."

It is an old saying that knowledge acquired without guidance goes haywire. The preceptor kindles the soul in you and is the dispeller of darkness (ignorance). Hence 'Guru' means one who dispels the darkness of ignorance and imparts supreme knowledge. A Guru is akin to a boat that is helpful to cross a river and a Guru helps us to cross the ocean of life to eternity.

15.3. Guru's guidance

This cosmic energy therapy is best effective when learnt from the lips of the Guru. This explains the old saying, "Unlinked grace of God will follow suit when guided by a Guru." The aspirant should be bestowed with the total grace of the Guru.

"No Guru's guidance = No God's grace"

Everyone cannot attain the supreme status of a Guru. Only a competent Guru can guide an aspiring candidate to perfection. An incompetent Guru falls by his own demerits. An anecdote from the Ramayana, perhaps, can throw much light. Sage Viswamitra takes Lord Rama with him to the forest to protect his penance from the disturbing interference and atrocities of Thaadagai, an ogress, who constantly engages in disturbing the sages, saints and their holy ritual observances. Sage Viswamitra tells Rama:

"O Rama! Kill that Ogress immediately!" But Rama is hesitant and asks the sage, "O venerable sage! Is it not a sin to kill a woman?"

Sage Viswamitra beautifully explains thus:

"If any sin strikes out of killing this ogress, let it strike me as you are killing her only on my direction. It is not prudent to punish the arrow when the person who shot the arrow is elsewhere".

Hence it is imperative that if a Guru misguides the aspirant, the sin accrued punishes the Guru himself, not the aspirant. **15.4. A Guru presents himself to**

an aspirant on the aspirant's merit in previous lives

It is customary in India to fall at the feet of the Guru to seek his blessings. Hence only a competent Guru, a realized soul, can adorn the role of a preceptor or a teacher or a religious head to perfection. When an aspirant falls to seek blessings at the Guru's holy feet, he gets up a new person, surrendering wholly of his sins at the Guru's feet. Only those equipped to vanquish those sins can become a Guru, or else the sins surrendered by the aspirant shall destroy the Guru himself.

As mentioned earlier, a competent Guru presents himself to an aspirant only based on the aspirant's merits accrued in a person's births. Hence saluting a Guru should be preceded by a careful analysis of whether he is qualified enough to be venerated. Saint Thirumoolar declares:

"Kurutinai Neekum Gururai Koallaar
Kurutinai Neekka Gurumai Kolvaar
Kurudum Kurudum Kurutaatum Aadi
Kurudum Kurudum Kuzhivizhum Aarea"

15.5. Knowledge is blind sans a Guru

For this cosmic energy therapy, recitation of holy incantations becomes necessary, which requires proper initiation from a Guru. Thirumandiram, composed by saint Thirumoolar declares:

"Guruvin Uruvum Kuriththa Appadhe
Thirumoolum Thirundhu Sivanavanaamea"

"When a guru is approached for guidance, the aspirant's sins are vanquished and he becomes eligible for God's grace." Though recitation of holy incantations does bring result, a Guru's guidance becomes all the more important for effective results. This explains why the scriptures declare that, "knowledge acquired without a guru's guidance is blind"

15.6. Composure is attained by uttering Guru's Holy Name Let us see the serene qualities of a Guru. A personification of all divine qualities, a Guru is a beacon light to ultimate wisdom. Only a person with a clear vision can guide another person.

In this context, this knowledge of cosmic energy can be best imparted only by learning from a Guru. Approaching a competent Guru and seeking this knowledge of cosmic energy begets positive results. But what is the essence of a Guru? Saint Thirumoolar explains:

"Thelivu Guruvin Thirumeni Kandaal
Thelivu Guruvin Thirunaamam Seppal
Thelivu Guruvin Thiruvaarthai Kettal
'Thelivu Guruvuru sindhitthal thaanea."

The term Guru means a very responsible position. The meaning of the explanation by the saint is as follows:

"You attain serenity on beholding the Guru's personality; You obtain tranquility on chanting Guru's nectar name; You bequeath all knowledge on hearing Guru's supreme utterances; And you reach the pinnacle of realization on contemplating the Guru's omnipotent form."

It is often said, "Sishya Paavam Guru Vimosanam."

Being in a responsible position, a Guru is held responsible for a sishya's mistakes. Utilizing this great responsibility with utmost care and acumen, it is the duty of a Guru to discharge his function to impart knowledge and guide the yearning souls to realization.

Saint Maanikavasagar was bestowed with the Supreme guidance of God Himself in human form as Guru. Irrespective of the age factor, anyone competent enough to teach the other can adorn the role of a

Guru. Lord Muruga, though very much younger to Lord Siva, assumed the role of a Guru and was celebrated by the devotees as Thagappan Swami (the God who taught his own father).

Hence, a Guru is one who dispels our ignorance, vanquishing our sins and rejuvenates our birth to the levels of sanctity. Only persons equipped to dispel one's sins should be venerated by falling at their feet. All of us should understand the difference between falling at a Guru's feet, which is nothing but absolute surrender of oneself completely to him, and falling at our elders' feet, which is an exhibition of the degree of respect we have for them and to seek their blessings soaked with love and care. An understanding of this difference becomes imperative.

15.7. Guru – A Beacon Light

As already mentioned, a Guru is a beacon light that guides an aspirant to wisdom and enlightenment. The following story is a testimony to this:

King Pariksheet attained realization by listening to the holy scriptures of Srimad Bhagavatam from a competent Guru. On hearing this, a jealous king desiring to obtain the same realization as that of king Pariksheet consulted many Gurus and studied the Bhagavatam. But the desired realization did not dawn on him. The king grew angry and consulted his minister. The minister, unable to find an answer to the king's question, excused himself promising an answer the next day. The minister was utterly confused. How can he cite a convincing answer to the king for not getting realization even after reading the Bhagavatam?

Seeing her father's deep concern, the minister's daughter came forward to answer the king's question. She approached the king and requested him to order everyone to leave the royal kingdom. The king agreed.

Now the minister's daughter requested the king to tie her to a pillar and then to tie himself. The king did so. After this, the minister's daughter now requested the king to untie her. The king was confused and said, "How can I untie you, when I am myself tied with the ropes?"

The minister's daughter, expecting this answer to drive home her point, replied: O king! This is the same state my father, your minister, is in now. How do you expect an ordinary man like my father to enlighten you on those aspects of knowledge that can be imparted only by a competent Guru? King Pariksheet's Guru is the storehouse of knowledge. Hence, that king was bestowed with the Supreme Knowledge when he listened to the Bhagavatam from the lips of such an extra-ordinary Guru. O! King! Understand that only a lighted lamp can lit another lamp. After all, my father is an ordinary minister seeking jewels and money from you. How can he answer your subtle question on enlightenment when he himself is not enlightened?

15.8. To Understand Truth and Untruth

In today's world, we witness so many so-called masters claiming their school of thought as the supreme among other theories. Let us reaffirm the truth, the only truth, that "God alone is Supreme." If the teacher is competent enough, then the aspirant will be benefited even without any practice. Such teachers existed before, not now. But even those aspirants, who had benefited from such teachers without enough practice, were matured souls. All that they required was the grace of Guru, on receiving which they attained realization.

Adoption and practice of cosmic energy therapy equips the aspirant to understand what is truth and untruth. The underlying working force of cosmic energy lies in channelising this energy by combining it with the grace of God.

I taught this cosmic energy therapy to a high-ranking officer in Chennai. But the officer did not believe in this simple technique of just placing the hand and approached another master. After a few days, he again returned to me, not to learn the technique but to hand over the course materials and the audio cassettes provided by that master to practice his technique. The officer was highly disturbed and went away and never came again. To tell the truth, no one believes the truth. Just like the omnipotent God who is found everywhere in the simplest form possible, the cosmic energy, too, is the simplest form of therapy that can be practiced and implemented to effective use, anytime, anywhere and by simple methods.

15.9. Guru, a Guiding Light

A Guru transforms the aspirant and elevates him to a higher position by infusing cosmic energy into him. As the very term Guru means Light, the hitherto hidden brightness of the aspirant is brought out by the Guru. A man in the darkness of afflictions, diseases and blockades is guided by the Guru to the light of good health, prosperity, and Supreme Knowledge. That is to say, the Guru dispels the tri-factors of arrogance, pride and illusion, imparts Supreme Knowledge and emancipates him to higher planes. This initiation, as it is known, is a sacred ritual, a ritual by which I channelise the cosmic energy through my head to my hands, infuse it to the aspirant's body, clearing the blockades and negative factors found in him. In simple terms, I am transferring the Buddha in me to the Buddha in the student. The divinity is passed on to the student, which is experienced blissfully in him. We can associate with another person when we transform him to the circumstances, efficiency and mode of level of communication to our level. In the words of the Sufi philosophy, the ultimate level of man's growth is his transformation into a good person.

15.9.1. Who are Eligible to Learn Cosmic Energy Way of Life?

Everyone can learn this cosmic energy way of life. Neither the learning demands a particular level of spiritual attainment, nor does it involve years of practice and training. This is an art of curing others, which does not depend on the individual's power. The cosmic energy passes on from the master to the student and consequently the student is also empowered with the cosmic energy. This qualifies the student to heal others. Simple and safe, this therapy can be imparted on anyone, an adult or a child.

15.10. A Modern World's Deceit!

Today's scenario is witnessing a plethora of commercial masters who claim themselves to be saviours of the worried. Combining psychology with spiritualism, they lure the youngsters to approach them. Oblivious of the trap set, these youngsters shun ancient methods as a mere gimmick and shell out thousands of rupees and dollars on these fake healers. Further, attractive advertisements mislead these youngsters into believing these so-called healers.

15.11. Modern Masters

These modern masters know the formula for deceiving the modern, educated public. They mix psychology with spiritualism, apply ineffective methods and offer a package, of course, with a heavy price tag attached to it. Even the modern youth are unable to decipher the truth and get deceived by these imposters.

An old film song comes to my mind, "Irukkum Idathai Vittu Illaadha Idam Thedi, Engengo alaigindraar Jnana Thangamae, avar edhum ariyaaradi jnana thangamae."

"O my lovable one! These people go in search all over, oblivious to its existence very near to them. I pity these people who are ignorant of this truth, O my lovable one!"

In this age of umpteen problems, both at psychological and physiological levels, the common man yearns for a quick solution. He is stripped of his commonsense and intellect by the attractive marketing strategy of these modern gurus and adopt their theories expecting short-term gains. These people have no idea whatsoever about the potency of ancient rituals, and never hesitate to shun them as baseless and unsuitable to modern times. Further, the apparently scientific observations and explanations of these gurus convince the common men that they are best suited for their spiritual and worldly developments.

A modern guru's luring dialogue:

"An ordinary man cannot control another man's mind. To achieve this, only I can, with my new-found vibrations from a new world".

15.12. Where is Peace, I want a Place There

"Peace cannot be bought," but people cannot accept this truth. Rich people do not mind shelling out big money to attain peace, but the poor cannot even afford to consult these rich gurus. But who cares for the poor? These gurus are content with the distribution of so-called books to reduce stress and win peace by charging Rs.1000 to Rs.2000 per session. These books brought by the gurus are nothing but a combination of the knowledge found in the Indian Vedas, Upanishads, and other books authored by leading writers on the subject. This practice of presenting others' ideas in a nutshell under the guise of their individual name cannot go on for long. This reaches a saturation point where both the aspirant and the so-called guru cannot understand or offer any new effective idea on their own.

This explains why people aggravate their grievances further, lured by the ineffective ways advocated by these socalled masters of modern age.

15.13 Beware of those who constantly mislead the People

It has now become very imperative to discriminate and be aware of some who indulge in intellectual discourses soaked in anecdotes from the history, quotes from the scriptures and interesting fables and tales to suit their theories.

Poet Pattukottai Kalyanasundaram beautifully says:

"They hail the law, standard of living and conscious appeals. O Fellowmen! Beware of these intellectually appealing speakers for it is an effective disguise to lure the public in the most modern terms."

As the popular proverb declares: "We can't cheat all the people all the time, we can cheat some people for some time only."

15.13.1. Maintain Distance – The Art Long-forgotten

Half the problems faced by the people will be solved if we could distinguish between the bad and the good. Poet Bharathi says beautifully:

"Nenjil Uramindri Nermai Thiranumindri Vanjanai Solvaaradi Ivar vai sollil veeraradi."

There is a group in this world that is highly moneyoriented and always indulges in deceiving people to make money. These people also find mean ways to make money like trying their luck in lotteries and other forms of gamble. As a shortcut to earn money, they accept bribes in their offices, only to be caught by law. Lamenting after all this cannot be akin to being wise. Hence, refrain from all these avoidable problems and adopt a natural way of life to live happily forever.

15.14. Holy Plates that Bring Luck

Many people fall for this trap of holy plates and ropes offered by money-minded individuals. If a good man with good thoughts gives these holy ropes, there is enough reason to buy them. But when one buys the same from fake individuals? Accepting these is only a sign of sheer stupidity. Hence, refrain from these useless practices that are both scientifically and spiritually baseless.

15.15. How to Identify the Right Guru?

The best judge is intuition. If you feel that a particular person is not worth going to, don't go to him. Else, follow the following tips that may reveal who is worthy or not. Those who claim these following declarations are not worthy of even a visit.

1. My method is the most potent of all.
2. My method encompasses all powers.

3. I am the only one to be initiated by the most powerful

Conclusion

Thank you again for downloading my book!

I hope this book was able to help you to learn about chakras.

The next step is to practice balancing the chakras for a balanced well-being.

I hope you enjoyed reading this book as much as I enjoyed writing it!

Thank you!

www.ingramcontent.com/pod-product-compliance
Lightning Source LLC
Chambersburg PA
CBHW072011070526
44583CB00015B/1432